OF PLAGUES
AND VAMPIRES

OF PLAGUES
AND VAMPIRES

Believable Myths and Unbelievable Facts
from Medical Practice

DR. MICHAEL HEFFERON

WOODPECKER LANE PRESS

ISBN: 978-0-9940172-8-4
Legal Deposit second quarter 2017
Library and Archives Canada, Ottawa

Library and Archives Canada Cataloguing in Publication

Hefferon, Michael, 1953-, author
      Of plagues and vampires : believable myths and unbelievable
facts from medical practice / Michael Hefferon.

Includes bibliographical references.
ISBN 978-0-9940172-8-4 (softcover)

      1. Medical misconceptions. 2. Medicine, Popular. I. Title.

R729.9.H64 2017   610   C2017-901249-5

Cover design: Maureen Garvie/ Allan Graphics
Author photo: Greg Black Photography

Typeset and printed by Allan Graphics Ltd.

Published in Canada by Woodpecker Lane Press
Kingston, ON   K7K 5E2
woodpeckerlane@gmail.com

CONTENTS

WE ARE WHAT WE EAT

MEDICAL CONTROVERSIES

A POTPOURRI OF MEDICAL MYTHOLOGY

PREFACE AND ACKNOWLEDGMENTS

SHAVING WILL MAKE YOUR HAIR grow in thicker. Swim right after you eat, and you'll get a cramp and drown.

True? Or only myths?

Myths, defined as "widely held but false notions," continue to pervade our everyday life. And after 40 years of practising medicine on three continents, I maintain that no group can hold a candle to medics when it comes to holding dubious beliefs, many of them propagated by our own profession!

When I entered medicine in 1970, Latin was a prerequisite, and biology was not. Extra points were given for classical Greek. Trinity College in Dublin graduated doctors with a combined degree in literature and medicine. But while medicine is rooted in ancient knowledge, it has been transformed, particularly since the latter half of the twentieth century, into a science-based medium for advancement of wellness and elimination of disease. In recent years, technology and bioscience have enabled medical scientists to prove or disprove beliefs that have been around for many generations.

Over the course of my 40-year medical career, 30 years of it devoted to the care of sick children, I have had countless encounters with beliefs closer to folklore than fact or science. For example: women have one rib more than men. Or: we should all be on gluten-free diets. Vampires really exist as a medical phenomenon. Electric shock treatment (ECT), rather than a tool in helping patients with mental illness, is a form of medical torture.

Treating a sick or troubled child today requires more than just lab tests and referral letters. One of my first questions is "What do the patient and the parents *believe* regarding their medical situation?" What if parents believe that a glass of wine the mother drank when she was pregnant caused their child's developmental symptoms? What if they believe that blood transfusions are likely to lead to permanent damage or infection to their child? Or, in the case of Jehovah's Witnesses, that the receiving of blood is damaging to their child's soul?

In these pages I explore these and many more beliefs. Join me in touring the interface of traditional beliefs as they meet modern medicine. And remember that in 1500 AD, professing a belief that the world was round rather than flat could lead to imprisonment, excommunication, or worse!

I am eternally grateful to all who encouraged and supported me in the writing of this book. Such an endeavour encompasses stories from teachers in my distant past and students in my day-to-day life.

Thanks to Midia, for your patience and endless typing.

To Catherine, Kate, Barry, and Claire for your special interest and help with the project.

And especially to Maureen Garvie, who has done so much to bring this book to its completion.

Michael Hefferon
2017

INTRODUCTION

I WASN'T LONG INTO my career as a physician and educator before I realized that many of my referrals were coming from colleagues, usually family medicine specialists. They often seemed uncertain as to the veracity of their own teaching on matters of childhood medicine. Does teething really cause fever in infants? Do iron drops really cause constipation in children?

At medical seminars — known as CMEs, for Continuing Medical Education — I developed a format I called "Pediatric Myths and Old Wives' Tales," which seemed popular with attendees. Many in my audiences were family doctors or nurse practitioners; all were interested in the true facts around common health problems.

Does covering our ears in cold weather help prevent ear infections, for example? Is acne caused by not washing one's face enough or by eating too much chocolate? Is gout, as many believe, the result of a lavish lifestyle of wine, women, and song?

We cling to our myths. It is hard to blame people for adhering to traditional folk remedies that appear to work, if we wait long enough. Homeopathy evolved in the 1800s; today, it is sometimes viewed as pseudoscience. However, back then, medics bled and leeched and purged people, performing primitive operations using whiskey as an anaesthetic. Some patients survived, and some were even cured.

Much of western medicine is built on concepts and practices arising out of the Greek and Roman cultures — cultures known for embodying their insights in myth. In classical Greek, the word *mythos* means story, while *logos* means something for which truth can be demonstrated. So, *mythology* translates as a story that is demonstrably true. Examples of myths with respectable connections to the medical profession are still with us; they include the Greco-Roman myths about Narcissus, Oedipus, and Ondine.

Narcissus was the son of a river god, who rejected the advances of a nymph. She then prayed to Venus, the goddess of love, who condemned Narcissus to an eternity of falling in love only with himself. Today we apply Narcissus's name to the term narcissistic personality disorder to describe a specific psychiatric diagnosis. These are people who lack empathy and have a deep need for admiration, along with an inflated sense of their own importance. Like Narcissus, they are in love with themselves. Sound familiar?

Oedipus in Greek mythology was a king of Thebes who, despite his own efforts to the contrary, fulfilled the prophecy of the Oracle at Delphi. He unwittingly killed his father, then married his mother, and with her produced four more children. In modern psychiatry, sexual attraction to one's mother has been given the name of "Oedipus Complex" — Sigmund Freud's theory on the various ways that children identify with the parent of the same sex, which, when unresolved, is a possible cause of a personality disorder.

Ondine was a nymph who wedded a mortal named Palemon. When Palemon was later unfaithful, he was cursed by Ondine to breathe only while awake, and so never slept again. The myth still gives its name to a medical condition known as "Ondine's curse" — a syndrome of "central apnoea" after spinal surgery, whereby patients can only breathe while awake and need ventilators to breathe while sleeping. Fortunately, neurosurgery patients with Ondine's curse can take a low-pressure ventilator home and sleep while the machine supports their breathing.

Today, myth is considered inferior to evidence-based science. The Oxford dictionary defines myth as "a widely held but false notion" — yet we have often heard that "myth is more potent than reality." What people believe is central to their upbringing, central to their culture and their experiences; it is influenced by their parents, teachers, clergy, and colleagues. Is that why myth continues to play such a significant role in medicine?

How many of the stories that surround us in the field of medicine are really myth, in the sense of "widely held but false," and how many have a scientific basis? Do some notions widely thought to be medical myths actually have some relation to fact? Let us explore the interface where a number of our traditional beliefs about health meet evidence-based medicine.

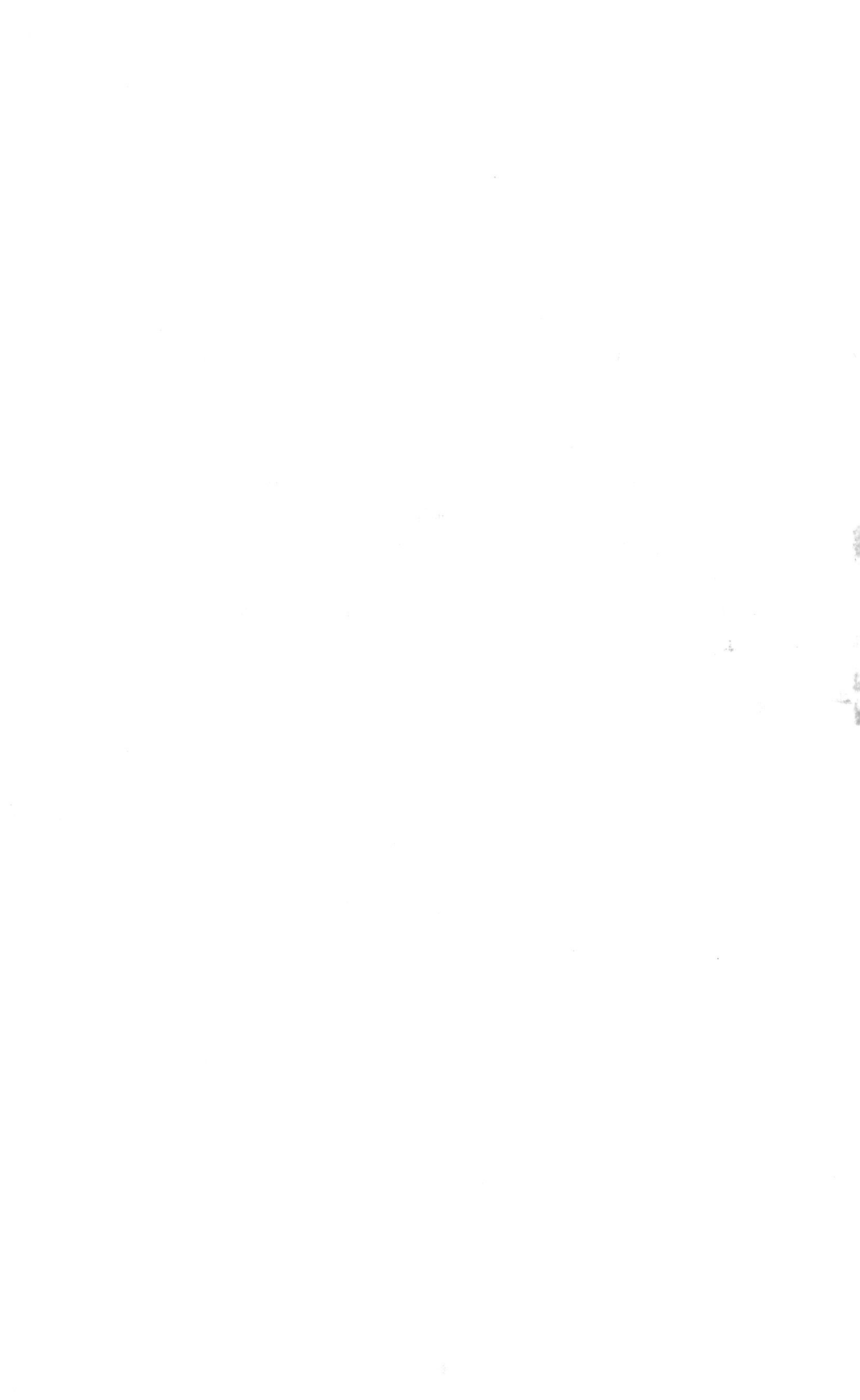

ANCIENT TRADITIONS

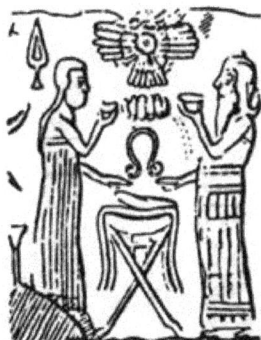

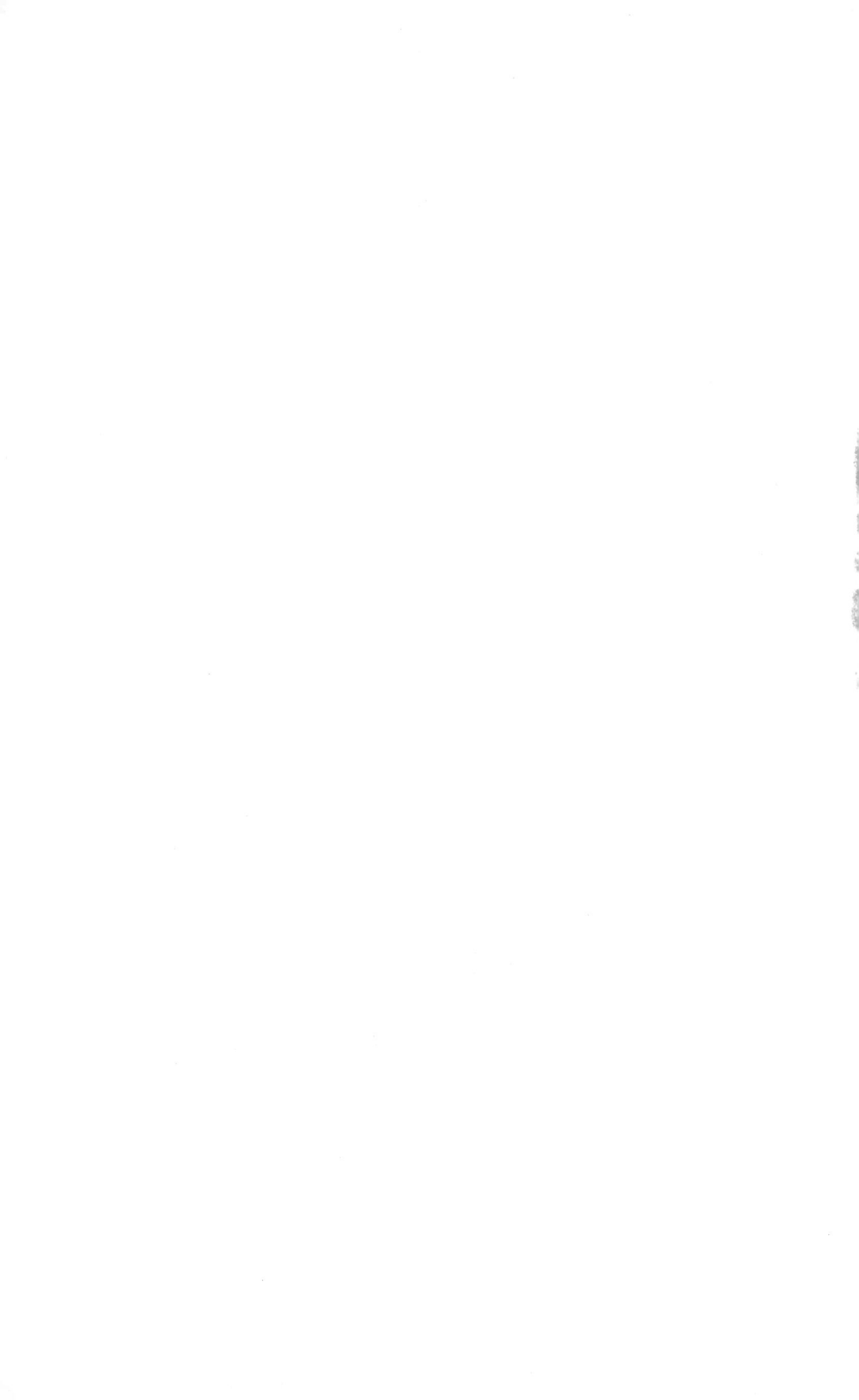

1 VAMPIRES:
ANY MEDICAL BASIS FOR THE MYTH?

THE CONCEPT OF A VAMPIRE predates Bram Stoker's tale of Count Dracula — probably by several centuries. Did vampires ever really exist?

In 1819, 80 years before the publication of Stoker's *Dracula*, John Polidori, an Anglo-Italian physician, published a novel called *The Vampire*. However, Stoker's novel has been the benchmark for our descriptions of vampires. But how and where did this concept develop? It appears that the folklore surrounding the vampire phenomenon originated in that Balkan area where Stoker located his tale of Count Dracula.

Stoker never travelled to Transylvania or any other part of Eastern Europe. (The lands held by the fictional count would be in modern-day Romania and Hungary.) The writer was born and brought up in Dublin.[1] He was a friend to Oscar Wilde and William Gladstone. He was both a liberal and a Home Ruler — in favour of home rule for Ireland. He turned to theatre, and became business manager of the Lyceum Theatre in London. It was his friendship with Ármin Vámbéry, a Hungarian writer,

---

[1] Stoker's younger brother, Dr George Stoker, emigrated to Montreal, where the family established roots in Canada, mainly in Quebec but later in Kingston, Ontario. George's great-grandson Dacre Stoker would one day write *Dracula the Un-Dead*, a sequel to Bram Stoker's novel.

that led to his fascination with vampire folklore. He consulted Vámbéry in the writing of *Dracula*, whose main character was loosely fashioned on Vlad the Impaler.

But where did the myth of vampires come from? Like many myths, it is based partly in fact. A blood disorder called porphyria, which has been with us for millennia, became prevalent among the nobility and royalty of Eastern Europe. A genetic disorder, it becomes more common with inbreeding. Porphyria is a malfunction in the process of hemoglobin production. Hemoglobin is the protein molecule in red blood cells that carries oxygen from the lungs to the body tissues. It seems likely that this disorder is the origin of the vampire myth. In fact, it is sometimes referred to as the "Vampyre Disease."

Consider the symptoms of patients with porphyria:

- *Sensitivity to sunlight.* Extreme sensitivity to sunlight, leading to facial disfigurement, blackened skin, and hair growth.
- *Fangs.* In addition to facial disfigurement, repeated attacks of the disease results in gums receding, exposing the teeth — which look like fangs.
- *Blood drinking.* Because the urine of persons with porphyria is dark red, folklore surmised that they were drinking blood. In fact, some physicians had recommended that these patients drink blood to compensate for the defect in their red blood cells — but this recommendation was for animal blood. It is likely that these patients, who only went out after dark, were judged to be looking for blood, and had fang-like teeth, led to folk tales about vampires.

- *A version to garlic.* The sulfur content of garlic could lead to an attack of porphyria, leading to very acute pain. Thus, the aversion to garlic.
- *Reflections not seen in mirrors.* In the mythology, a vampire is not able to look in a mirror, or cannot see their own reflection. The facial disfigurement caused by porphyria becomes worse with time. Poor oxygenation leads to destruction of facial tissues, and collapse of the facial structure. Patients understandably avoided mirrors.
- *Fear of the crucifix.* At the time of the Inquisition, it is reported that 600 "vampires" were burned at the stake. Some of these accused vampires were innocent sufferers of porphyria. Porphyria patients had good reason to fear the Christian faith and Christian symbols.

Acute attacks of the disease are associated with considerable pain and both mental and physical disturbance. This condition has been ascribed to the English King George III, although subsequent analysis has shed some doubt on porphyria as the cause of his "madness."

Nowadays, with our scientific knowledge of the basis of porphyria, instead of fearing these folks, we can love and care for them. Porphyria remains incurable, and treatment is mainly supportive: pain control, fluids, and avoidance of certain drugs/chemicals that provoke acute attacks. Some success has been achieved with stem cell transplants.

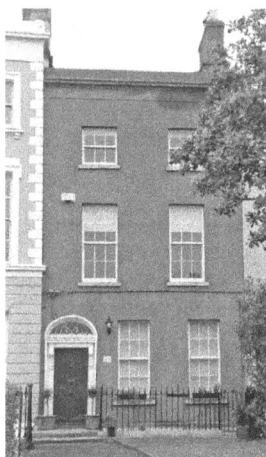

Stoker's birthplace, Marino Terrace, in Dublin

Could Stoker have known of the existence of the medical condition of porphyria, and of its link to vampire folklore? It was only in 1911, eight years before Stoker's book appeared, that a German physician, Hans Gunther, classified the diseases of porphyria (there are several types). However, George Harley, of Harley Street, had described a patient with porphyria a few years earlier.

Through his gothic novel, Bram Stoker surely wins the prize for the best example of myth entangled with medicine!

REFERENCES

Murray, P. From the shadow of Dracula: A life of Bram Stoker. Random House, 2004.

Gueco, M. Porphyria, the vampire disease that started the legend. KNOJI- Knowledge. 2009. https://knoji.com/porphyria-the-vampire-disease-that-started-the-legend.

Hift, R.J., T.J. Peters, P.A. Meissner. A review of the clinical presentation, natural history, and inheritance, of variegate porphyria: Its implausibility as the source of the "Royal Malady." J ClinPathol, 2012, pp. 200–205.

Dundra, G. Porphyria and the folkloric vampire. BMJ, 1999, pp. 319–335.

2 LEPROSY:
A PIECE OF HISTORY, OR STILL A THREAT?

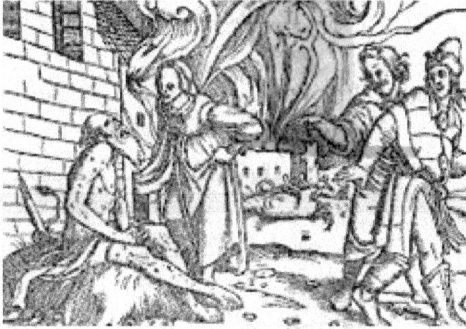

LEPROSY IS A DISEASE known to us since biblical times. But have you known or known of anyone with this disease?

Are there still leper colonies?

In the Bible (Luke 17: 11-19), Jesus encounters ten men known as "lepers." Historically, lepers were forbidden entry to towns and were required to ring a bell, announcing their contact risk. Jesus cures the men, and the priests in the town certify them as "clean." Only one man, however, returns to thank Jesus.

Leper colonies, or quarantine houses, were common in the Middle Ages, often run by religious missionaries. Leprosy was greatly feared because of the disfigurement and disability that it causes.

Despite its biblical descriptions, leprosy is not highly contagious. It is most likely transmitted by the respiratory route from untreated individuals, usually over long-term contact. While the disease usually starts with a characteristic skin rash, it goes on to damage the nerves in the fingers and toes. The lack of sensation leads to skin damage and numbness, resulting in tissue loss. It also leads to paralysis of small muscles.

Leprosy is today known as Hansen's Disease, named after Armauer Hansen, a Norwegian doctor who in 1876 first observed under a microscope the bacterium Mycobacterium leprae that causes the disease.

The cure came in 1950. Dr. Vincent Barry, in Trinity College, Dublin, while working on medications to counter tuberculosis, stumbled on Dapsone, an antimicrobial that was discovered to be effective against the leprosy bacterium. That discovery was to save 15 million lives. Dapsone, in combination with other anti-TB drugs, is still used to treat leprosy.

Spinalonga in Crete was one of the last leper colonies to close, in 1957. However, if we reflect on the fact that HIV has been largely contained, and that 65 percent of people with cancer now beat it, it is incredible to learn that leprosy is still infecting people. United States has 100 new cases of leprosy each year. In 2013, in the state of Maharashtra, India, 35 new cases presented to one clinic alone in a one-week period. In the same state, it is documented that 5,000 people have been cured of the disease and now live on in relatively good health.

So, while it's a myth that leprosy has been eradicated, it is also a myth that it untreatable and irreversible. Leprosy can now be cured.

REFERENCE

Yadav, N., S. Kar, B. Madke, D. Dashatwar, N. Singh. Leprosy elimination a myth busted. Journal of Neurosciences in Rural Practice, vol. 5, suppl. 1, 2014, pp. 28-32.

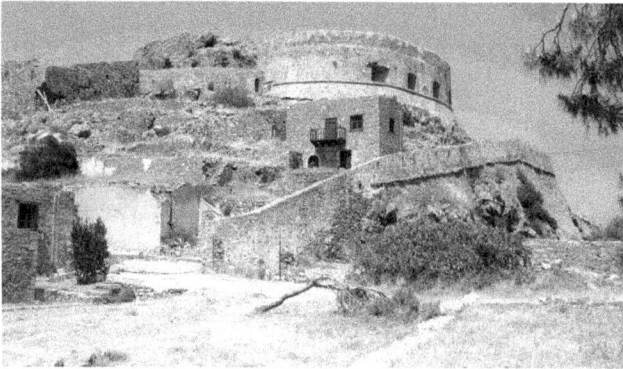

The former leprosy colony on Spinalonga Island, Crete

3 DIVINE INTERVENTION: CAN PRAYER EFFECT MEDICAL OUTCOMES?

MANY OF US HAVE family or friends who have faith that praying at a time of misfortune, surgery, or life-threatening illness will improve the outcome. Some researchers have attempted to find if this is actually the case.

Difficulties arise when scientific analysis is compared with theological arguments. The scientist first needs to assume or prove that God exists, that prayer can travel through space to reach God, and that God is responsive to prayer and can influence the outcome for the better. Theological arguments will be based instead on certainty that God exists, is receptive to prayer, and has omnipotent ability to influence outcomes through a mechanism unknown to science.

To study the efficacy of prayer, medical science would require performing trials that were randomized and double-blinded. Subjects would be picked at random, and the patients would have to be unaware of whether they were being prayed for or not. Then, for a further period, the roles would have to be reversed, with the original group proceeding without prayer while the other group was prayed for, at a time of great medical concern. Not an easy job to do, and for sure no one has done it.

However, studies have been done in randomized fashion, and ten of these studies were analyzed by the *Cochrane Review* to report on what evidence could be found. The

Cochrane Review is an international organization that reviews human research and reports in an evidence-based fashion. In 2009 the review looked at ten randomized trials which it felt tested the hypothesis that "praying to God can help those who are prayed for." The conclusion was that the methodology of these trials can scarcely allow outcomes to be presented as proof. They also beg the question as to whether God would intervene in case A and ignore the plight of case B.

The studies fail as well to address the controversy as to whether death is necessarily always a negative outcome. For instance, if a very elderly person has a debilitating stroke, perhaps that person should be allowed to depart this world and not linger in pain.

Some of the prayers in the studies were actually retroactive, with prayers coming after the event. (Analysts pointed out that there was no *time* in heaven.)

One trial showed a small reduction in deaths from sepsis (blood infections) in those who were prayed for. Another study found an actual increase in surgical complications in the prayed-for group, but only if they *knew* that they were being prayed for.

One study in Korea at an IVF clinic reported that prayer could be related to success rates in pregnancy. The prayed-for group had a better pregnancy rate. However, the prayers were exclusively Christian, and many in the study were Catholics, whose church is opposed to IVF. Is this outcome therefore a positive one?

In summary, the *Cochrane Review* felt that the mixture of science and theology was unsound in all ten studies and that much additional research was needed.

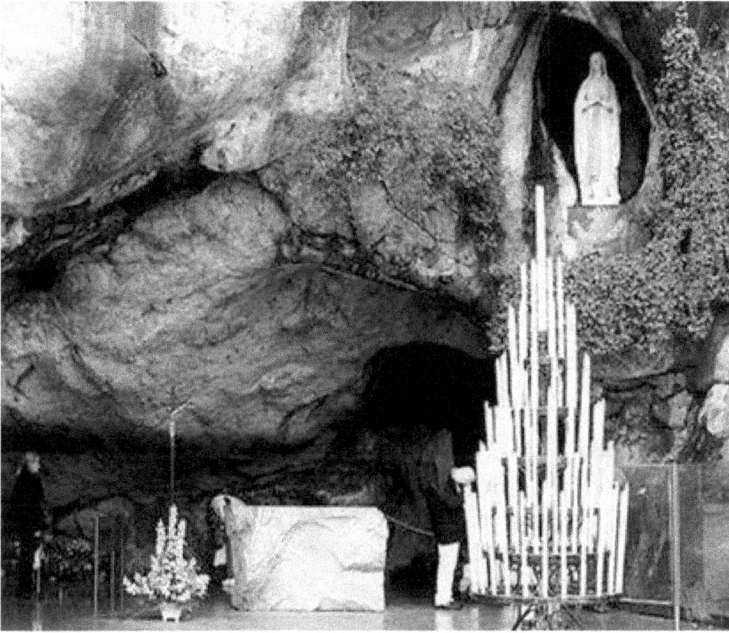

The Grotto at Lourdes, site of 67 verified miracles

Perhaps it would be better to have atheists conduct these studies to remove bias. Certainly, a science-based model is needed before we can conclude whether the claim of improved outcomes from prayer for the sick is a myth.

However, this is not to say that prayer and religious faith do not benefit persons diagnosed with serious disease. Researchers looked at coping strategies in elderly women recently diagnosed with breast cancer. They concluded that 91 percent reported that religious faith provided emotional support; 70 percent reported strong emotional support; and 60 percent felt that religion now brought meaning to everyday life.

These effects could of course be related to faith and social support rather than divine intervention. So ... come back in 30 years!

REFERENCES

Jørgensen, K.J., A. Hróbjartsson, P.C. Gøtzs. Divine intervention? A Cochrane Review on intercessory prayer gone beyond science and reason. *Journal of Negative Results in Biomedicine*, 2009, p. 7.

Feher, S., and R.C. Maly. Coping with breast cancer in later life: The role of religious faith. *Psycho-oncology*, vol. 8, no. 5, 1999, pp. 408-416.

4 EPILEPSY: OLD DEMONS
OR NEW UNDERSTANDINGS?

MY DOCTOR, MY FRIEND, my neighbour, my favourite musician, and my local police officer all have it. Add to the list Charles Dickens, Vincent Van Gogh, Alfred Nobel, Richard Burton, Julius Caesar, and Sir Isaac Newton, and you may realize how pervasive this condition is. Today there are some 50 million people with epilepsy worldwide.

One seizure does not constitute epilepsy. Epilepsy is a disease involving *recurrent seizures*. The origin or cause of these neurological episodes is unknown in the majority of cases, rendering it a primary disorder (a condition not known to be related to other medical pathology).

Epilepsy may be the most misunderstood and stigmatized condition in human medicine. In the twenty-first century, the lore and beliefs of our past seem hard to change. Even the term epilepsy comes from the Greek verb *epilambeneim,* meaning to be seized, or taken by surprise.

As historically all diseases were regarded as a form of punishment, this condition was regarded as a form of retribution. Sufferers were believed to be possessed by demons. The ailment was thought to be infectious, and thus isolation was employed. The first enlightenment came with Aristotle, who felt it was an organic disorder. It wasn't until 1875 that an English neurologist described it as a disruption in electrical activity in the brain. In 1930, a device called the *electroen-cephalogram* first recorded electrical activity from the brain and allowed objective diagnosis.

The first anticonvulsant (bromide) came to us in 1875. Now dozens of such medications control seizure activity and allow for a more normal life. However, one-third of patients still have poorly controlled (refractory) epilepsy.

And not all persons who experience seizures are only mildly impaired. Persons with neurological disorders have a higher incidence of seizures — for instance, 25 percent of children with cerebral palsy have accompanying seizures. Many of these seizure patterns can be severe, depending on the degree of neurological damage.

But a large number of healthy functioning children and adults have not been permitted to take part in mainstream society as a result of mythology. Some of this stigmatization is compounded by inaccurate portrayals of epilepsy in the media:

- Demonic possession. (Remember *The Exorcist*?)
- Foaming at the mouth. This rarely happens in a seizure and is merely a stereotype.
- An object must be placed in the patient's mouth to stop them swallowing their tongue. This is not the right thing to do, and no one can swallow their tongue.
- People become violent in a seizure. Patients are unconscious and unable to demonstrate violence.

It is also sometimes believed that persons with epilepsy have lower IQs. This myth is based on the fact that school leavers with epilepsy often demonstrate poor academic achievement. However, this may relate to several factors other than IQ. For instance:

- Confusion and memory loss are common after a seizure.
- Absence seizures (petit mal) may be mistaken for daydreaming.
- Drug therapy: Many anticonvulsants slow cognitive function and interfere with short-term memory.
- Children with seizures may miss more school or be stigmatized by seizures in the classroom.

The stigma of epilepsy is often more disabling than its neurological effects. I quote Orrin Devinsky, a landmark American neurologist: "For persons with epilepsy, fighting the stigma of cultural bias is followed in life by educational underachievement, low self esteem, restricted opportunities for social activities, poor employment opportunities, and problems with intimate relationships." These negative attitudes to epilepsy can lead to difficulty in finding employment and developing relationships. Vulnerability in social situations, where a seizure can occur without warning, leads to withdrawal from society, further compounding the problem.

Equal-opportunity employment bodies and epilepsy societies have done Trojan work in advocating for persons with epilepsy. Increasing awareness among employers, schools, and career guidance officers has moved this cause forwards.

Up to now, people with epilepsy have been reluctant to disclose their condition when applying for jobs. However, employers and colleagues might well consider learning what to do in the event of a seizure. Epilepsy also affects what insurance is available for the employee and the employer. Clearly there are some jobs that will not be open to people with epilepsy in the interest of safety. For instance, in Ontario one needs to be seizure free for six months to drive a car. In the United States, one needs to be ten years' seizure free (without medications) to have a commercial driver's licence.

However, being employed gives people a sense of identity and self-worth and provides structure in their day, while helping them to be viewed as valued members of society. It can be hard when these doors are closed.

The fact that society in general is 50 years behind the times in awareness of epilepsy truths is a fixable problem. Consider this: the year I entered medical school in 1970 was the year that the UK law prohibiting marriage of persons with epilepsy was repealed. That would hardly have done a lot for intimate relationships in former years!

When we consider the opinion of a neurological surgeon, Dr. Joseph Price, who stated in 1892 that the causes of seizures lay in "debauchery, chocolate, coffee, excessive lust, and amorous love songs," I suppose we have come a long way.

REFERENCES

Baxendale, S., and A. O'Toole. Epilepsy myth alive and foaming in the 21st century. Epilepsy and Behaviour, vol. 2, no. 2, 2007, pp. 192-196.

Price, J. The surgical treatment of epilepsy. JNervMent Dis., 1892, pp. 396-407.

Maria, S.L., and O. Devinsky. Epilepsy and behaviour: A brief history. Epilepsy and Behaviour, vol. 1, no. 1, 2000, pp. 27-36.

Voskuil, P.H. The illness of Vincent Van Gogh. J HistNeurosci, vol. 14, 2005, pp. 169-175.

5 THE ROD OF CADUCEUS:
ONE SNAKE OR TWO?

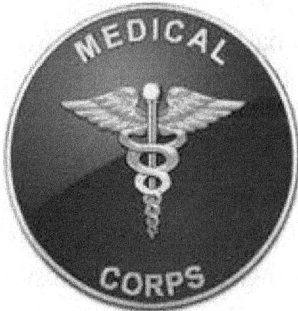

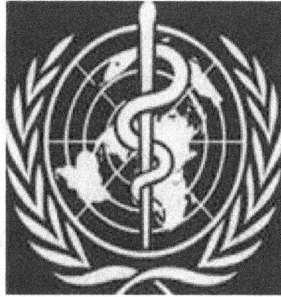

THE SYMBOL ON THE LEFT above is probably familiar to you as the symbol of medicine or healing. It is common to see this symbol in North America, since the Caduceus was adopted by the U.S. Army's Medical Department at the beginning of the twentieth century.

The rod stands for power, the serpents stand for wisdom, and the two wings represent diligence and activity. However, this emblem is actually the symbol of Hermes, the Greek god who is protector of merchants — and tricksters and thieves!

The symbol on the right, the Rod of Asclepius, is the true symbol of medicine and healing. It is the symbol adopted by the World Health Organization and all national medical organizations. Unlike the Rod of Caduceus, it has only one snake and no wings.

Asclepius was a Greco-Roman god of healing, worshipped as the son of Apollo. Historians have traced his existence to the sixth century BC. He was perceived as a patron of physicians and as the origin of the rod of physicians. His daughters are Hygieia, goddess of hygiene and cleanliness, and Panacea, goddess of remedies.

The origin of this symbol is also fraught with myths. One story tells of Asclepius treating a patient who was threatened by an approaching snake. He killed the snake with his staff and retained it as a symbol of healing.

So, how much do most doctors, nurses, or medical students know about this symbolism of their profession?

In 2014, a study was undertaken of 200 doctors and 100 medical students to assess their knowledge of medical symbols, among them the emblem of healing. Only 6 percent of doctors were aware of the rod of Asclepius as the true emblem of healing.

Humans are fond of symmetry, and so many may simply find the symmetrical Caduceus more attractive than the Asclepius. Many institutions continue to use the Caduceus rather than the Asclepius as their symbol, and that is unlikely to change.

REFERENCE

Shetty, A., S. Shetty, O. Dsouza. Medical symbols in practice: Myths vs. reality. Journal of Clinical Diagnostic Research, vol. 8, no. 8, 2014, pp. 12-14.

6 FEVER THROUGH THE CENTURIES

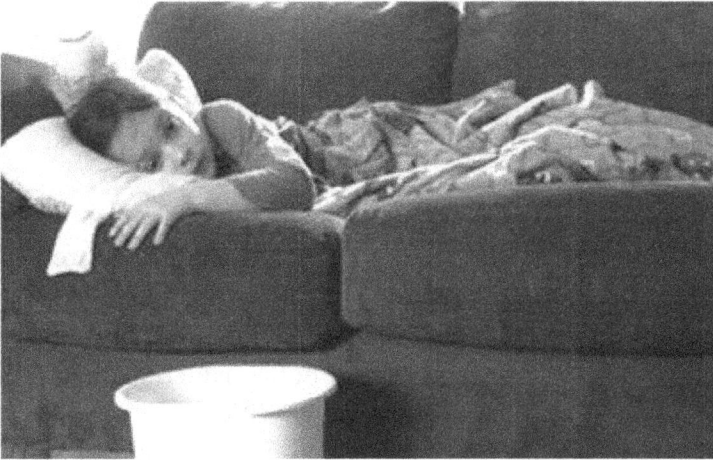

PROBABLY NO OTHER medical topic is as fraught with myth as fever, particularly fever in children. Partly to blame is that the causes of fevers may range from inconsequential to life-threatening.

Even the definition of fever varies widely. Fever is generally agreed to be *an elevation in body temperature above the normal range.* But what is a normal body temperature? In general, you could take 37 degrees Celsius as a normal body temperature and 38 degrees as a fever. However, this range varies over the journey from the cradle to the seniors' home.

It isn't valid to report a temperature based on a flushed infant with a warm forehead. Temperatures are measured at many body sites. Generally speaking, core body temperature, measured in the rectum, is 0.5 degrees higher than a measurement taken peripherally, such as under the armpit. Some medical practitioners may even ask for a correction for the time of day, believing the afternoon body temperature to be 0.5 degrees higher than one taken later in the day.

Most people do not have baseline measurements of their own normal body temperatures. As these vary, it might be possible to entertain different definitions of fever for given individuals.

Fevers account for 30 percent of children's medical visits and 20 percent of all emergency room visits. These figures demonstrate the magnitude of the clinical problem. It is unlikely that any other single issue reaches the significance or volume of this complaint. "Fever phobia" is ascribed to parents who are unduly anxious about the possible outcomes of fever in their children. However, fever phobia is also found in nursing staff and medical staff.

Fever anxiety is usually related to adverse experiences of children with fevers, or reports they've heard about negative outcomes. Dismissing fevers would be foolhardy. Fever in an infant under two months of age is more likely to be a manifestation of serious bacterial infection than fever in a six-year-old. Also, fever in an unimmunized child requires a different set of considerations from those of a regular fever visit.

So, armed with this introduction, let's look at some of the myths that have developed over the centuries, many of which are still around.

Does serious infection always manifest as fever?

While fever is a common manifestation of infection, not all serious infections will have a fever at examination. The most sinister example is a child in septic shock. In this condition, bacteria invade the bloodstream in large numbers and cause a clinical state of *shock*. The result is low blood pressure and poor blood supply to the skin and vital organs. In this scenario, the temperature measurement will actually be low, not high — a state called *hypothermia*. This condition is fatal unless treated quickly and aggressively. Even with treatment, morbidity and mortality are significant. This outcome is probably the number 1 reason for fever phobia and for the enormous number of visits to doctors and emergency rooms. The infection may start with fever, but in the shock stage there will be no temperature elevation.

The higher the fever, the sicker the child?

One of the most benign conditions in pediatric medicine is called roseola. This is a viral illness caused by human herpes virus type 6. The infant will usually have an extremely high temperature, often 40 degrees, but no other findings are evident, and all x-rays and blood tests are normal. Then, after three days, a characteristic rash declares itself, and all is well again. However, the rash does not appear until after the three days of high fever.

Fundamentally, if the child looks sick, the event is serious. People can look well with a high fever, and paradoxically, can look ill with a low-grade fever.

What does "looking ill" entail? Ask any parent. A child who is lethargic, uninterested in activity or fluids, and exhibiting unusual behaviour is far more likely to need medical attention than a child with fever alone.

The longer the fever, the more serious the disease?

Generally speaking, a febrile (showing symptoms of fever) illness in a child or adult will resolve in three to four days.

If a serious condition is neglected, symptoms will persist until the correct treatment is implemented. But what about fevers that continue for five days, two weeks, or more? Does the length of a fever indicate a more sinister outcome? The answer is usually *yes.* Below are three scenarios in which prolonged (or recurrent) fevers are likely to be significant.

Kawasaki disease : Mainly a viral illness of children, the hallmark of Kawasaki disease is a fever that lasts five days or longer. It would be unusual for influenza, ear infection, or tonsillitis to last this long, particularly with treatment.

Kawasaki disease is far from benign. Accompanied by a characteristic rash, conjunctivitis, and peeling of skin, this illness can attack the coronary arteries and lead to heart failure and long-term heart complications. It is treated with intravenous protein antibodies.

Collagen disease : This term encompasses a group of chronic conditions such as rheumatoid arthritis, lupus, and scleraderma. These are often life-long debilitating diseases that can cause multi-organ damage. And often they start with a fever.

Persistence of the fever into a second week should alert medical caregivers that infection is not the only origin of fever. Persisting elevations of certain inflammatory markers will guide doctors towards a collagen diagnosis.

Malignancy: Rarely, a malignancy may be the cause of fever in a child. While we regard cancer as rare in children, it is not totally unusual, and leukemias, lymphomas, and solid tumours are known to present with fever.

Doctors are sometimes obliged to exclude cancer as a cause of prolonged fever even though it is only likely to be the case for a tiny fraction of the total number of children with fever.

In most of such instances, fever is a minor accompanying sign rather than a major presenting sign. Fever will not resolve until the malignancy is treated.

Periodic fever syndrome

Recurrent fevers without identifiable causes need to be investigated thoroughly. But what if, after multiple exhaustive tests, no cause is evident, and the fevers recur at intervals of weeks?

A condition called PFS, a genetic disorder, is still incompletely understood. Children with PFS develop sporadic fevers starting in infancy. Tests are negative, and the fevers run a generally benign course. It's common for their parents to tell the doctor that in childhood they themselves were "fever babies" — a term used in generations past for this condition. The genetics are now more clearly understood.

Familial Mediterranean fever is the most common of these PFS conditions. It is found in people of Mediterranean ethnicity and has been identified as MEFV gene. A defect in this gene will lead to poor control of inflammation and to spontaneous fevers that are not infectious.

While there are a few other genes whose defects cause PFS, the above condition is the most common. Although these children are not infectious, daycares and schools are often concerned that they aren't safe for other children to be around. In fact, they pose no danger.

Are fevers above 40 degrees dangerous? Can they lead to brain damage?

While very elevated temperature readings are uncomfortable for patients and frightening for caregivers, it is a myth that they are going to cause brain damage — or any damage, for that matter. Fever is the body's response to an inflammatory trigger such as a virus or other infection. Fever helps the body to fight infection.

Within the context of an illness, fever will not rise above 42 degrees. However, there are other situations that can cause body temperature to rise to levels that would damage brain function. The two main triggers for this are:

1. Extreme environmental temperatures, such as a child being locked in a car in hot weather.
2. Malignant hyperthermia, a condition of genetic origin triggered by certain anaesthetic agents, wherein muscle metabolism runs amok, and overwhelms the body's capacity to regulate body temperature. Lab studies are unreliable in identifying susceptible individuals. The best preventatives are to avoid dangerously high temperatures and causative anesthetic agents (for example, by proper flushing of anaesthetic tubing).

Can children with high temperatures have febrile seizures?

It's a common myth that untreated fevers result in febrile seizures. In fact, studies have failed to show any relationship between the onset of seizure activity and the height of the fever.

Despite the horror of witnessing a child in a febrile seizure — a simple short seizure in a child from six months to six years old — the evidence suggests that the outlook for normal brain function is excellent.

Simple febrile seizures occur in approximately 4 percent of children. (Complex febrile seizures last longer than 15 minutes and often occur in children with pre-existing neurological damage.) Some children will have multiple recurrences of seizure with fevers; 33 percent of children having febrile seizures will have more than one.

The origin of this lowered seizure threshold seems to be genetic. Families will frequently report a history of other members experiencing these events.

Recovery is rapid and complete, and CT scans and MRIs are not indicated. The vast majority of these children will subsequently have a normal EEG (brain wave test).

Do all fevers need to be treated?

As fever is actually beneficial to the body's immune system, it is really a symptom and not a disease entity. One might argue that *not* treating it might be beneficial to the patient!

However, febrile illnesses come with a significant degree of discomfort, which probably justifies relief of symptoms. The medical profession generally agrees with the following advice:

1. Fevers up to 38.5 degrees Celsius should be left untreated.

2. Above 38.5 degrees, it is reasonable to give symptom treatment, usually repeated every four hours.
3. Giving fever-lowering agents will not prevent febrile seizures.

Feed a cold and starve a fever?

We can trace this "wisdom" back to England in 1574, when a man called John Withals published a dictionary in which he advised that "fasting is a great remedie of feuer."

Back in the 1500s, the cause of "colds" was not known and was blamed on a drop in body temperature. Eating food was thought to help the body generate warmth during a cold, while laying off calories helped cool the fever's heat. Perhaps this was the start of the chicken soup routine.

Who knows? How easy would it be to conduct an experiment to validate this claim? Well, one group of lab scientists in Holland have had a go. At the academic medical centre in Amsterdam, a group of healthy individuals were put through periods of nutrition and alternating starvation. After each exposure, the lab analyzed immune response factors in blood samples. There were significant boosts to immune protein levels in both situations, but different immune proteins were involved in feeding and fasting.

In scientific terms, food intake stimulates levels of gamma interferon, while food deprivation stimulated interleukin-4 release. Both proteins are involved in helping the immune system in different ways.

Could it be that John Withals was right all along?

REFERENCES

Perry, A.M., A.C. Caviness, J.Y. Allen. Characteristics and diagnoses of neonates who visit a pediatric emergency centre. Pediatr emerg care, no. 1, 2013, pp. 58-62.

Walsh, A., and H. Edwards. Management of childhood fever by parents. J Adv Nurs., vol. 54, no. 2, 2006, pp. 217-227.

Spruijt, B., Y. Vergouwe, R.G. Nijman, M. Thompson, R. Oostenbrink. Vital signs should be maintained as continuous variables when predicting bacterial infections in febrile children. J Clin Epidemiol, vol. 66, no. 4, 2013, pp. 453-457.

Verity, C.M., and J. Goldring. Risk of epilepsy after febrile convulsions: A national cohort study. BMJ, vol. 303, no. 6814, 1991, pp. 1373-1376.

Withals, J. A dictionary for young beginners. British Museum Library, 1574.

7 IS SHOCK TREATMENT STILL USED TO TREAT MENTAL ILLNESS?

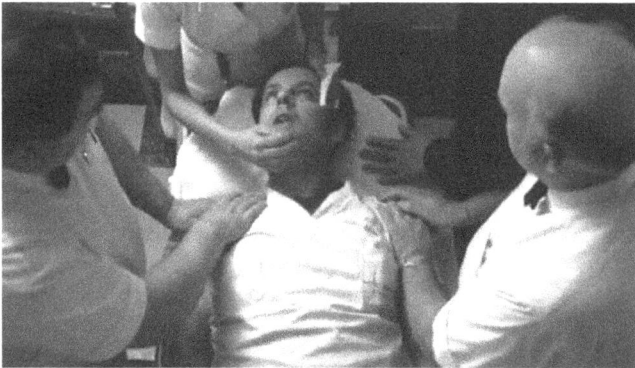

FOR MOST PEOPLE, it may be a shock to hear that electro-convulsive therapy, or ECT, is still in use.

Many of us recall the memorable 1970s movie *One Flew over the Cuckoo's Nest* where the inmate troublemaker was given ECT as a punitive measure. The image of a reluctant, terrified patient strapped down to have shock treatment administered seems still to be all too common. Thus, it may be surprising to learn that 100,000 people in the United States receive ECT each year, and some receive ECT regularly, even several times a week.

ECT was introduced in 1938 for the purpose of inducing convulsions in patients to relieve severe depression and psychosis. After media portrayals of the treatment as violent and inhumane, its use declined in the 1960s with the arrival of effective antidepressant and antipsychotic medications.

Despite the historical horror associated with this treatment, updated studies do confirm the effectiveness of ECT for many patients. The Cochrane database reviewed 26 trials and 50 reports of ECT, compared to placebo or "sham ECT" (when patients are prepared with anaesthetic as if for ECT but no current is passed). The studies confirm a lower rate of relapse after ECT.

While the reasons that ECT works are not fully understood, we do know that in some cases urgent resolution of symptoms is necessary — for suicidal patients, for example, or for those with severe schizophrenia that is unresponsive to medication. Make no mistake, the treatment induces a seizure in patients. However, treatments are not always given in a mental institution and can actually be delivered on an outpatient basis. You can look at it as "rebooting the system" — turning the computer of the brain off and on again.

ECT is not barbaric or dangerous. Patients are given general anesthetic and a muscle relaxant before the treatment. They do not break teeth or bones during the procedure. The treatment has rapid results in 85 percent of cases. However, some patients experience memory loss in the hours or days following treatment.

ECT is not a cure for anything: it is just another treatment. One reason that we don't see much use of ECT today is that it is labour intensive and expensive to deliver, particularly when compared to prescription medications or even psychotherapy.

Most people can be well managed with these treatments and do not need ECT.

So think of ECT not as a punitive horror but as a more humanized treatment of last resort, which improves quality of life for many people for whom other treatments have been ineffective.

REFERENCES

Tharyan, P., and C.E. Adams. Electroconvulsive therapy for schizophrenia. Cochrane Database SystRev, January 2005.

Payne, N.A., and J. Prudic. Electroconvulsive therapy, part 2: A biopsychosocial perspective. J Psychiatr Pract, vol. 5, 2009, pp. 369-390.

Leong, O.K. Myths and realities of electroconvulsive therapy. Singapore Med J., vol. 34, no. 3, 1993, pp. 262-264.

MYTHS OF A GENDERED PERSUASION

8 WOMEN LIVE LONGER THAN MEN: OR ARE TIMES CHANGING?

NEXT TIME YOU HAVE reason to visit a seniors home or an assisted living facility, have a look around. Yes, there are more women than men — but how many more? The truth is, that for every 100 men aged 85 and over, there are 425 women. Some facilities even advertise a "women only" policy and have no shortage of applicants.

It's hardly news that in western society, men have a higher mortality rate than women up to age 85. Through history, this disparity has been taken for granted, with very few conversations around the topic. After all, the male bee dies after mating, sacrificing himself for another generation. And throughout history men have died in wars, many never seeing their offspring grow up.

Recent generations have blamed the higher mortality on a twofold elevation of arteriosclerotic heart disease in men. Why so?

- Men have traditionally smoked cigarettes more than women. Thus, they experience more deaths from lung cancer and emphysema.
- Aggressive and competitive behaviour, which is stressful, is considered a male trait. Guns, fatal

accidents, cirrhosis, and hazardous jobs all pertain more to a male culture than a female one.
- Female hormones may have a protective effect. For example, coronary artery disease is uncommon in women of childbearing age.

So, why was I condemned at birth to die three years before my female neighbour? If the reason were that men were physically stressing themselves through work into an early grave, then we would be seeing a narrowing of the gap, as today many men and women do similar jobs. However, this three-year age expectancy gap has remained consistent. In regions where men smoke and drink more (e.g., Russia), men die 13 years earlier than women. But natural history teaches us that among our closest primate relatives, chimpanzees and gorillas (who do not smoke or drink), females still consistently outlive the male of the species.

The answer probably lies in the hormone testosterone deemed responsible for maleness — a deep voice, a hairy chest, and aggression. So what if males were to live life with little or no testosterone? The imperial court of the Chosun Dynasty in Korea kept eunuchs to guard the royal harem. Castrated before puberty, they had an average lifespan of 70 years at a time when the average male in the court lived only to 50.

Not only are females protected by not having testosterone but they may also be protected by estrogen, which acts as an antioxidant and protects cells from stress. This female advantage in survival is called the "longevity gender gap," or LGG. This advantage is seen in almost every country in the world, with the exception of Sardinia, which has no LGG. No one has managed to explain why this is so.

There may also be a further protective effect from women having two X chromosomes, allowing for an extra copy of many genes, which may work as "spare parts" in a stressful lifespan.

Whatever we believe about the origins of LGG, it is a myth that men are going to catch up with female longevity anytime soon.

REFERENCES

Austed, S. Why women live longer than men: Sex differences in longevity. Gender Medicine, vol. 3, no. 2, 2006, pp. 79-92.

Poulain, M., G. Pes, L. Salaris. A population where men live as long as women: Villagrande Strisaili, Sardinia. Journal of Aging Research, 2011; ID 153756.

Kirkwood, T. Why women live longer than men. Scientific American, April 1, 2015.

9 SHOULD A SURGEON BE CALLED DOCTOR, MISTER, OR MS?

IF YOU'VE HAD OCCASION to meet a male British surgeon, you will notice that his title is Mr. Smith, not Dr. Smith. If you worked for such a surgeon, you would not call him Dr. Smith twice. Some women who have joined the ranks of surgical dissectors have chosen to be called Ms. Smith.

So why would a student become a physician after seven long years and then proceed with a further seven years of apprenticeship of the most rigorous kind, only to return to his or her common name? Sharing the title of Mr. or Ms. with the butcher and the baker does not sound like the surgeons you know. What could be behind it? History, dear folks, history.

Centuries ago, surgeons were not considered qualified enough to call themselves "Doctor." So when they were finally offered the title, they refused it on principle!

Have you ever wondered why a barber shop has a red and white flagpole outside, looking like a candy cane out of season? The history that lies behind it is that barbers in medieval Europe were surgeons. They performed surgery — including bloodletting, draining abcesses, extracting teeth, and, of course, cutting hair. The red and white striped pole was meant to reflect the blood and the strips of bandages involved in the surgical procedures.

Most of these "surgeons" were illiterate, without medical training. Surgeons were not admitted to a physicians' guild. Then, in 1745, King George II founded the London College of Surgeons. By 1800, the guild had been granted a royal charter and became the Royal College of Surgeons, as distinct from the Royal College of Physicians. Surgeons at this point had medical training: all medical practitioners, whether physicians or surgeons, had to undertake training at medical school to obtain a qualifying degree. Yet the tradition in Britain of a surgeon being referred to as Mr./Miss/Ms./Mrs. has continued, meaning that in effect a person starts as Mr./Miss/Ms./Mrs., becomes Dr., and then goes back to being Mr./Miss/Ms./Mrs. again!

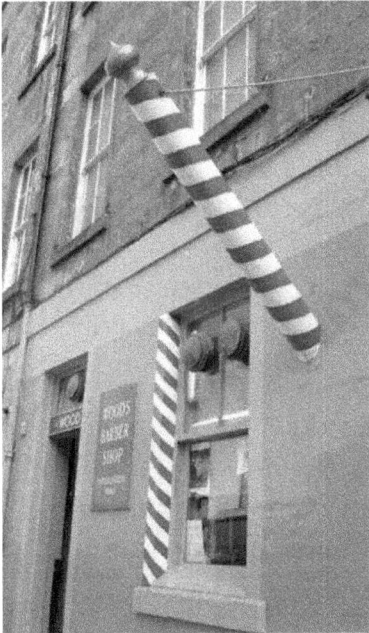

Traditional barber-shop pole

In North America there is no such historical distinction. In Canada, the two disciplines have always been combined in the Royal College of Physicians and Surgeons. So a surgeon in Canada or United States still wants to be addressed as "Doctor" and does not relinquish this title on receiving a fellowship in surgery.

How do you distinguish physicians and surgeons? Often you don't. In Ontario, all surgeons are called "Doctor" and their ID tags say "Physician" — to the chagrin of surgical staff who come to Canada from the UK.

How long will this hierarchical title last? Maybe not that long. In Australia, which carried this tradition far across the world, the Royal Australasia College of Surgeons is moving to establish "Doctor" as the universal title for surgeons. However, there is no such move afoot in the doorways of Harley Street.

REFERENCES

Pelling, M. Barbers and barber-surgeons: An occupational group in an English provincial town, 1550–1640. Bulletin of the History of Medicine, vol. 28, 1981, pp. 14-16.

Qualifications of a Surgeon. Royal College of Surgeons of England, Lincolns Inn Fields, London, WC2A 3PE.

10 FOR WOMEN, IS 40 THE NEW 20?

FOR A MAN, IT'S generally not an issue. The saying "A man is never too old" is legendary. Men do not experience menopause and, at least theoretically, remain fertile into late life. Les Colley, an Australian man, had a son at age 92 on January 1, 1998. Media sources claim that Ramajit Raghav, from Haryana in northern India, fathered a child at age 94 and again at 96.

And lately, pregnancies in women into the sixth and even seventh decade of their lives are no longer making headlines. But are we covering up uncomfortable facts about childbearing in later life?

The era of modern reproductive choices began in the 1960s with contraception and legalized abortion. Women could postpone pregnancy while they embarked upon careers. As a result, despite the falling birth rate over the past three decades, the birth rate among women aged between 35 and 55 has risen.

This rise is associated with upbeat media reporting of older women having babies, often through the use of reproductive technology (fertility treatment/donor sperm/donor eggs/ freezing eggs/IVF). These favourable reports have been based on small numbers and early results.

The media's positive portrayal of youthful-looking women balancing home life and career is well accepted. But as we age, we acquire medical conditions that can complicate pregnancy: for example, diabetes, hypertension, and risk of premature birth. So even with much popular support promoting motherhood and encouraging a level playing field for women, is 40 the new 20, reproductively speaking?

I recall when I was a resident in obstetrics that 29 was considered the peak age for childbearing — in other words, things were going downhill after age 29. Pregnant women were considered "elderly" at 35. We seldom saw pregnancies in women after 40, and if we did, it was seldom a primagravid (first pregnancy) and rarely a multiple pregnancy. Today the definition of Advanced Maternal Age has crept up to 40, and now the term "Very Advanced Maternal Age" is used for women over 45.

The choice to delay may also be a product of many young fertile women hearing their mothers or grandmothers describe how their aspirations in life were diverted by the arrival of a baby. Or many may feel that their partners are not ready to settle, despite the fact that women are most fertile between the ages of 15 and 30.

This is where the science kicks in. A woman's eggs are as old as she is. Whereas men make sperm every month or two, women are born with a full quota of eggs. Over time, then, as these eggs age, their chromosomes are less likely to divide properly (a condition called aneuploidy). The rate of aneuploidy by age 40 is 75 percent. The majority of fetuses with aneuploidy will abort spontaneously. But the incidence of Down Syndrome rises from to 1 in 400 with a mother in her early twenties to 1 in 60 at age 40. Incidence of other aneuploidies — Patau Syndrome and Edwards Syndrome, chromosome abnormalities not unlike Downs — increase twentyfold.

Yes, these concerns are reduced by the use of donor eggs, but such interventions do not guarantee a receptive uterus.

Although there is no current definition of advanced *paternal* age, studies are showing decreases of sperm quality and motility after age 35. As well, recent studies have indicated an association between autism and advanced paternal age.

Unfortunately, when sex-education classes discuss the deferral of pregnancy, childlessness and birth defects are seldom mentioned. But they should be. Older women can give birth to healthy children, but the chances get slimmer with time. So while the key to informed choice is education, we need to recognize that, as far as having babies is concerned, 40 is not the new 20 — despite what we may be led to believe.

REFERENCES

Dietl, A., S. Cupisti, and U. Zollner. Pregnancy and obstetric outcomes in women over 40 years of age. Gebertshilfe Frauenheild, vol. 78, no. 8, August 2015, pp. 827-832.

Delpisheh, A., L. Brabin, and B.J. Brabin. Pregnancy in late life: A hospital-based study of outcomes. J Womens Health, vol. 17, no. 6, July 2008, pp. 965-970.

11 GOUTY OLD MEN?

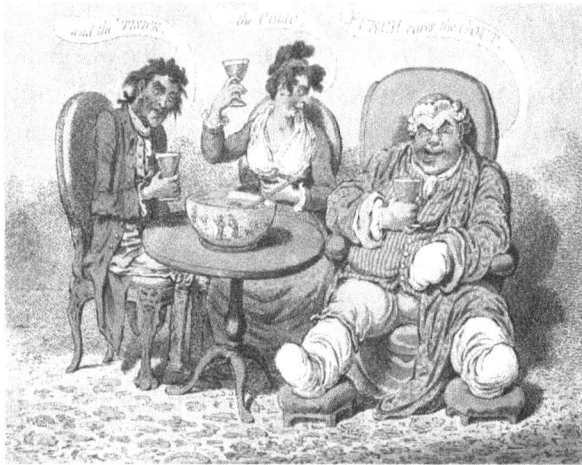

SO WHAT DID Henry VIII, Phillip II of Spain, and Luciano Pavarotti have in common? Beethoven and Leonardo da Vinci? Pitt the elder and Pitt the younger? You guessed right if you said they all had gout.

Although we have known about gout for at least 4,000 years, the stereotypic image of a Pickwickian older gentleman bingeing on port and Stilton has dominated society's image of gout. But what is true, and what is myth?

Gout has often been referred to as the "disease of kings" — Charles IV, V, and VII were all sufferers. But gout also afflicted Queen Anne of Denmark and Queen Anne Stuart of Scotland.

To get beyond the popular stereotype of persons with gout, it's important to know that gout is not a lifestyle disease but an inherited disorder of uric acid metabolism. Gout is in fact caused by uric crystals collecting around a joint, such as the big toe, and causing severe arthritic pain. Although the uric acid crystals were first identified as a cause of gout in 1859, it was not until 1988 that a Nobel Prize was awarded for the discovery of a medication (allopurinol) that would reduce the production of uric acid crystals.

Gout is the commonest cause of arthritis in men over 40, and as people are living longer, it's on the increase. By the age of 60, the incidence of gout in men and women is equal.

Most of us can eat, drink, and be merry without fear of developing gouty arthritis, but many people with gout are quite abstemious. It's not a complete myth that rich diet can be associated with gout, however. Beer, liver, and sardines are all very high in purines (a form of animal protein) and are hard to metabolize if you have a genetic deficiency of the enzymes that break down purines.

So people with gout do need to watch their diet — just like the rest of us.

REFERENCES

Rider, T., and K. Jordan. The modern management of gout. Rheumatology, vol. 49, no. 1, 2010, pp. 5-14.

Roddy, E., and H. Choi. Epidemiology of gout. Rheumatic Disease Clinics of North America, vol. 40, no. 2, 2014., pp. 155-175.

12 THE RIB MYTH: DO WOMEN HAVE ONE MORE THAN MEN?

HERE'S A PRE-MED exam question:

Is it a myth that women have an extra rib compared to men?

   a. Yes
   b. No
   c. Maybe
   d. Men have the extra rib
   e. None of the above

When this question is posed to medical trainees or even medical professionals, the instant reaction is hesitation. Somehow, our brains will jumble what we learn in the medical training with what we've heard early in life. This is more particular to those of us over the age of 40, and most of us who are from Judeo-Christian backgrounds. Younger folks, who are not as likely to be influenced by the Bible, are less likely to be confused on the topic. In Genesis 2:22, God takes a rib from Adam and makes a woman (Eve). This is the ancient story of creation in the Old Testament.

Darwin long ago provided us with a scientific alternative to creationism, and most people no longer adhere to the Adam and Eve story. But is there more to it than Genesis?

One day as I was spinning the rib myth for trainees in the paediatric common room, a young woman spoke up. "My mother has one more rib than my father. My sister also has an extra rib. Both have had surgery to remove it, and I'm being investigated myself for having an extra rib!"

Could this be? Three women in one family with an extra rib not found in male family members?

This young woman, a dietary intern who was rotating through Paediatrics that week, was describing a condition called Thoracic Outlet Syndrome caused by a cervical rib — indeed, an extra rib — in the neck area. The result is often compression of nerves and blood vessels coming through the neck into the arm. The condition affects 0.6 percent of the population, but females are affected three times more often than men. This would translate to 30 million females world-wide having an extra rib, and only 15 million males. And so, technically, it is indeed more common for a woman to have this condition, but it has very little to do with myth!

REFERENCES

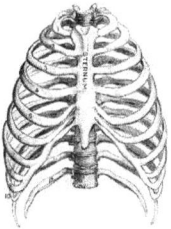

Genesis 2: 22: "Then the Lord made a woman from the rib he had taken out of man."

Dolansky, S. The immortal myth of Adam and Eve. https:// thetorah.com/the-immortal-myth-of-adam-and-eve/.

13 EQUAL SEX RATIO AT BIRTH?

ULTRASOUND NOW ALLOWS us to know the gender of a foetus after about 18 weeks of gestation. Boy or girl? The odds are 50:50 — right?

The answer may not be as obvious as the question. It's a myth that the actual sex ratio is 50:50. In developed countries, 105 boys are born for every 100 girls. In China, and in the East in general, the figure runs from 110 to 118 boys per 100 girls. (Chinese figures are affected by the preferential abortion of females and by the one-child law, but other eastern countries have higher ratios without these laws.)

Parental age (maternal and paternal) can cause a change in this ratio, with older parents being less likely to have a boy.

So why might all this be? Theories abound, but the following factors may be relevant:

1. A male foetus is less likely to make it to term. Intrauterine deaths are more commonly male, and survival in the pre-term infant is biased towards females. Therefore we could surmise that nature starts with an excess of boys for this reason. (Remind me again, which is the weaker sex?) However, advances in antenatal care in the past 70 years may have benefited male foetuses more than females.

We suspect that gender ratios at birth may have been 50:50 in the nineteenth century, when many of these male offspring were not salvageable.

2. Male offspring were more likely to be killed in war or in accidents, ending up with women outliving them in later life.

3. In pediatric practice, in the 1970s and 1980s, I recall many families with multiple children — indeed, it seems that fewer people had children, but those who did had *more* children. Also conspicuous was the observation that some large families had five girls, while other families might have six boys. The question arises: once you have a boy, are you destined to have more boys? Once you have a girl, are you more likely to have girls?

The situation is not so simple, but there are patterns that suggest that this may be more the case with boy babies. Allowing that your chance of conceiving and giving birth to a girl on the first try is 49.5 percent, if you go ahead and try for a girl after having one male child, your chances are 50:50, and after having two boys, this goes down to 47.7 percent. After three boys, that chance of having a girl falls to 43 percent. Not massive ratio changes, but significant in a world of over seven billion people.

4. The percentage of boys born increases during and after wartime. Why would that be? Did heaven replace the losses at the Somme with a male ratio imbalance? It's a fact that male births (and all births) spiked in 1857 (the Crimean War), 1919, and 1946.

The age of the mother at conception does not affect the gender of the child, but the age of the father does. Younger men are more likely to conceive boys.

Other theories suggest that tall men are more likely to produce boys. It's also true that taller men are more likely to survive war.

Put all this together, and consider that taller, younger men, returning from combat with burning passion, eager to be intimate more often, might do so at times in the cycle that would favour male embryo creation — mid-cycle — and these ratios are not hard to believe.

In conclusion, then, whether in war or peace, it's a myth to believe that the sex ratio of our babies is 50:50.

REFERENCES

Catalano, R., and T. Bruckner . Secondary sex ratios and male lifespan: Damaged or culled cohorts. School of Public Health, University of California. 2006.

Graffelman, J., and R.F. Hoekstra. A statistical analysis of the effect of warfare on the human secondary sex ratio. Human Biology, vol. 72, no. 3, 2000, pp. 433-444.

Bernstein, M.E. A genetic explanation of wartime secondary sex ratios. American Journal of Human Genetics, vol. 10, no. 1, 1958, pp. 68-70. PMID-13520702.

TERMINATING THE CANCER MYTH

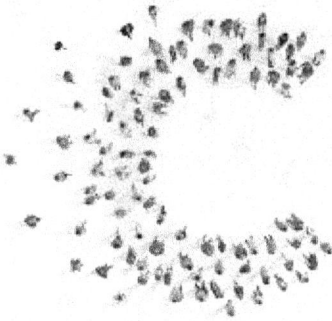

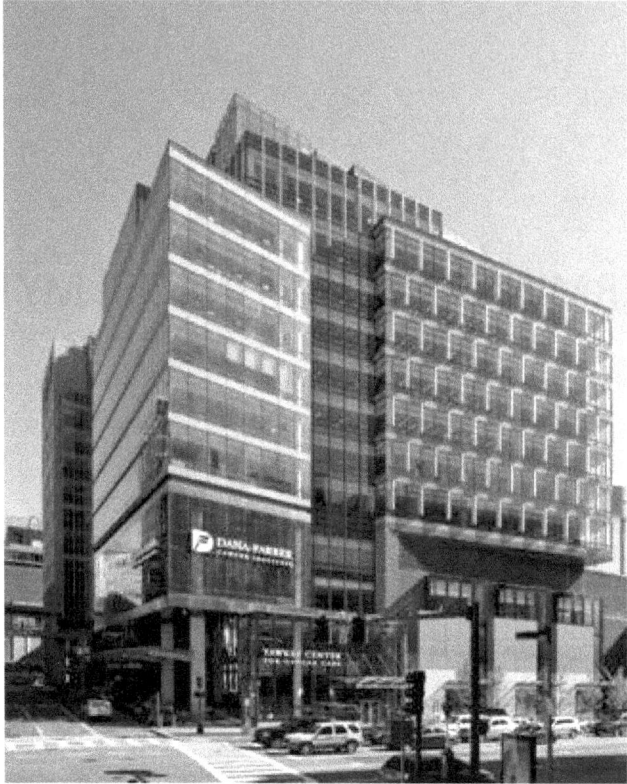

The Dana-Farber Cancer Institute in Boston

14 A VITAMIN CURE FOR CANCER?

THE BENEFITS OF VITAMINS have led to a multi-million dollar industry that has far exceeded the original intent of these products.

Vitamin deficiencies, particularly deficiencies in vitamin C such as scurvy and vitamin D such as rickets, were landmark discoveries in the progress of nutritional medicine. For instance, deficiencies in Vitamin B, which has 12 components including thiamine (B1), folic acid (B9), and cobalmin (B12), can contribute to problems from mood disorders to heart disease.

In the 1940s, there were popular theories regarding the benefit of vitamins for just about everything. In Boston, Dr. Sidney Farber was interested in blood disorders. He had seen the benefit of some B vitamins in treating pernicious anemia. Thus he set out to treat patients with childhood leukemia with Vitamin B9, or folic acid. These unfortunate children rapidly declined and died within weeks instead of months. The cause was that vitamin B9 was feeding the leukemia cells and actually helping the cancer (leukemia) cells to grow.

Dr. Farber set about finding an agent that would do the opposite — choke off the cancer cells. He teamed up with his laboratory to synthesize an "anti-folic acid agent" called Methotrexate. Methotrexate prolonged the children's lives, but it was 20 more years before the arrival of "combination chemotherapy," which resulted in significant survival of children with acute leukemia. Dr. Farber became known as the father of chemotherapy and has been honoured by the great Dana-Farber Cancer Institute in Boston, named for him with support from the Charles Dana foundation.

When I was a student in the 1970s, survival in acute leukemia in children was about 20 percent. Many of these children sustained life-long complications from chemotherapy and radiation. By the time I was a resident, this survival figure had risen to 40 percent. Still, many patients succumbed to complications and infections. In 2017, the long-term survival rate among girls with standard-risk acute lymphoblastic leukemia was 94 percent, with complications being rare.

So it was the discovery of an agent that would *block* a vitamin that resulted in the discovery of chemotherapy. And, in its time, this discovery almost did not happen. Sidney Farber was born in Buffalo in 1903 into a Jewish family. He was one of 14 children. In the 1920s, many Jewish students were refused entry to US medical schools on the basis of quotas. The Farbers spoke German, and Sidney found a place at the University of Heidelberg. Such was his success in that first year that he was admitted to Harvard as a second-year student.

REFERENCES

Simone, J.V. Fifty years in hematology: Research that revolutionized patient care. American Society of Hematology; 50th Anniversary Meeting, 2008.

Foley, G.E. Obituary for Sidney Farber. American Association for Cancer Research, vol. 34, 1974, pp. 658-661.

15 IS CHILDHOOD CANCER INCURABLE?

PERHAPS NO VISION in our media is more potent than that of a small child, left without hair as a result of cancer treatment. It's barely believable that life, or circumstance, or God, could be cruel enough to allow a young child to be diagnosed with cancer.

Many of these images are used to increase awareness of the terrible plight of these children, and their families. They are basically our neighbours.

And make no mistake, these images do raise awareness. Better still, they raise money. And that may be considered money well spent. Advances in care have benefited from research funding. Thankfully, expectations may now increase along with it.

So, how rare is cancer in children today? While we can hardly say that childhood cancer is common, it is the leading cause of death by disease in the developed world, in children aged two through 18.

This year, in Canada, there will be 2,000 cancer diagnoses in persons aged 18 and under. Approximately 80 percent of these children will survive their ordeal.

Thus comes a new cohort of survivors of childhood cancer, who need to be followed medically for the remainder of their lives. Many and most will lead normal, healthy, productive lives that would not have been possible a generation ago.

However, the medical follow-up is life-long. Although many people will encounter little or no long-term medical complications, some will have lasting effects from their disease and/or its treatment.

These late effects can depend on the type and location of cancer, the type and dose of chemotherapy, the child's age when treated, and any other health problems that may have existed before diagnosis.

Late adverse effects can include growth suppression, hormone and fertility problems, radiation toxicity, secondary (later) cancers, steroid toxicity, learning difficulties, and emotional problems. Complications, and after-effects from bone marrow transplantation, can also be significant.

In brief, there are three main types of childhood cancer (and many more types that are less common). These are acute leukemias, brain tumours, and lymphoma.

These three diagnoses account for the majority of cancers in children. (Others such as Wilms Tumour, a kidney malignancy, and neuroblastoma, a nervous-system tumour, are unique to pediatrics but are not as common as the first three mentioned.

So it comes as no surprise that the leukemias (cancer of the bone marrow, the spongy centre of bones that makes blood cells) represent over 30 percent of all childhood cancers. There are clearly high risk and low risk groups. The good news is that in the lowest risk group, a survival rate of 94 percent is now possible.

Through history, a survival of five years past diagnosis has been judged to be a cure. (This definition is not universally adhered to). More importantly, the *disease-free,* intact survival has massively increased. In children, this is important, as in the past the use of radiation was associated with disfigurement, particularly after spinal radiation.

The discovery that spinal radiation was not needed in milder cases of leukemia, and the more selective use of radiation with other tumours, has led to better outcomes with less or no disfigurement. How was this achieved? We need more than money, and goodwill to turn around such a plague. The answer is *collaboration.*

The Children's Oncology Group (COG) is a clinical trials group with more than 200 member institutions in United States, Canada, Australia, and New Zealand. The COG has enabled data from all regions of these countries to be assessed and outcomes to be compared, looking at the factors that may have affected outcomes in these children.

So it transpired that children on leukemia treatment in New York, Christchurch, and Kingston, Ontario, could receive the exact same treatment protocol, and that data during the course of treatment could be shared with other centres for the benefit of all. Not only were patient details shared and reviewed, but the events and responses to relapses were also shared. This collaboration led to a 44 percent reduction in mortality from relapse between 2000 and 2005.

Adults with leukemia do not fare as well as children. This is because adults tend to acquire a more aggressive form of leukemia.

Genetics and ethnicity may also affect outcome. This again relates to the sub-type of leukemia. For instance, in Canada, two-thirds of children will have the lower risk variety. In North Africa, the statistics are inverted, and two-thirds will have the higher risk type.

So these are meaningful gains and improvements in the lives and families of childhood sufferers. We also have some way to go. Our goal is 100 percent intact, long-term survival. The last part of this battle may be the hardest.

The caring, loving families of children with cancer will frequently ask us, "Can we treat her with *natural products*?" This question may reflect their fear of toxicity of chemotherapy agents. Perhaps they are partly correct. For now, though, we need to define what we mean by standard medical care and what we understand to be "natural medicine."

Standard medical care (also referred to as *mainstream medicine*) is medicine practised by health professionals who hold an MD degree. They are frequently joined by nursing specialists, called nurse practitioners.

Complementary medicine is a form of treatment used *along with* standard medical care. These are not standard treatments but could take the form of, say, acupuncture, to help lessen the pain of cancer treatments.

Alternative medicine is usually what people are referring to when they speak of "natural medicine." These are treatments that are used *instead of* standard medical treatments. An example might be using a special diet instead of chemotherapy to treat cancer.

Physicians are sometimes criticized for dismissing so-called natural therapies in favour of mainstream medicine. Commonly, I am asked, "But doctor, what harm can it possibly do?"

In the previous chapter I explained that Vitamin B (folic acid) can actually accelerate the course of cancer and result in early demise. The herb kava kava, used to reduce anxiety, can cause liver damage. St. Johns wort can interfere with the efficacy of some chemotherapy agents. We ask that patients inform us of any or all of the products and dietary supplements they are taking, so our pharmacists can check whether they could interact negatively with mainstream treatment.

Fundamentally, the word *natural* does not mean *safe*.

REFERENCES

Hunger, P., X. Lu, M. Devidas, B. Camitta, P. Gaynon, N. Winick, G. Reaman, W. Carroll. Improved survival for children and adolescents with acute lymphoblastic leukemia between 1990 and 2005: A report from Children's Oncology Group. J ClinOnc, March 2012.

Kaatch, P. Epidemiology of childhood cancer. Cancer Treatment Reviews, vol. 36, no. 4, 2010, pp. 277-285.

16 DOES WEARING SUNSCREEN PREVENT SKIN CANCER?

NOT ALL SKIN CANCERS are equal. To emphasize the differences, we talk in this chapter about melanoma skin cancer and non-melanoma skin cancer.

Malignant melanomas (MMs) make up only about 2 percent of skin cancers, and yet they are responsible for more than 80 percent of deaths from skin cancer, often following a change in a pre-existing mole. The past three decades have seen an increase in the incidence of melanoma in persons over 50. The incidence of the disease in younger people is stable, but people are living longer, and the incidences of all cancers are increasing in the older population.

The other types of skin cancers (non-melanoma) are less malignant and make up the other 98 percent of all skin cancers. They consist of basal cell carcinoma and squamous cell carcinoma. They involve more benign lesions and are related to prolonged sun exposure. While these lesions rarely progress beyond local skin lesions, some, especially squamous cell carcinoma (which are even less common), can spread to nearby tissues.

Genetics is known to play a role in the development of malignant melanoma. If you have a first-degree relative (a parent or sibling) with MM, the risk of your developing it is doubled. Certain genetic patterns are more commonly seen in people with MM. For instance, CDKN2A is a tumour suppressor gene that can undergo mutation (change) and allow the malignancy to occur.

Before we dig into micromolecular structures, there are very obvious patterns in the distribution of skin cancer that tell us more about its natural history. Malignant melanoma is 25 times more common in whites than in people of African descent. It is also less common in people who tan well. For instance, it is five times less common in Hispanic and East Indian folks than in Caucasians.

Evidence shows the role of sun exposure in the causation of MM to be "sun injury" — a bad sunburn — rather than sun exposure. Basal cell and squamous cell carcinoma are a feature of "prolonged sun exposure," not necessarily sun injury. Basal cell carcinoma tends to occur on each side of the nose and also at the tops of the ears — areas of maximum exposure. For that reason, many golfers concentrate their sunscreen on those skin areas.

So where do we find the biggest incidence of non-melanoma skin cancers? Wait for it: the top three countries are Switzerland, Ireland, and Canada (especially Manitoba). How does this make any sense, especially when the *lowest* incidence in the United States is in California? To further confuse you, California has a high population of Hispanics, but in fact it's the white population of that state that has the lowest incidence of skin cancer.

I can tell you personally, from 30 years living in each of Ireland and Canada, that exposure to the sun, let alone the appearance of the sun, can be a rare event. Manitoba has glorious winter sunshine, but I've yet to see people sunbathe in minus 30 degrees. So, if the cloudiest country in the world (Ireland, surely) has the second-highest incidence of skin cancer, surely more than just sunshine is to blame. It is conceivable that when the sun does shine, people are more prone to expose themselves to extreme amounts of sun over short periods of time.

Where does sunscreen come into the picture? Is it the answer to preventing skin cancers? Maybe not....

So far, sunscreen has not been shown to reduce the incidence of either melanoma or non-melanoma skin cancers. In fact, the availability of sunscreen has led to longer periods of intentional sun exposure, and more frequent sunburns. Over the two decades or so in which we have seen generalized use of sunscreens, the incidence of skin cancer has actually risen. This may go partway to explaining why MM is more common in indoor desk workers than in outdoor field workers!

In 1977, Bob Marley went to his doctor for removal of a wart on the undersurface of his foot. This wart turned out to be a malignant melanoma, which was to cause his death in 1981. Certainly, this was not due to sun exposure. Bob was also Anglo-Jamaican. His father was a British naval officer from Liverpool.

Melanoma can also occur in the rectum and in the vagina. Very confusing, isn't it?

It seems to be a myth that sunscreen is going to prevent deaths from skin cancer. We need to acknowledge, however, that even though people with an indoor lifestyle can die of skin cancer, sun damage frequently plays a causative role.

REFERENCES

Huncharek, M., and B. Kupelnick. Use of topical sunscreen, and the risk of malignant melanoma: Results of a meta-analysis of 9,067 patients from 11 case control studies. American Journal of Public Health, vol. 92, 2002, pp. 1173-1177.

Chestnut, C., and J. Kim. Is there truly no benefit with sunscreen use and Basal Cell Carcinoma? A critical review of the literature and the application of new sunscreen labelling rules to real world sunscreen practices. Journal of Skin Cancer, vol. 11, 2012.

Planta, M. Sunscreen and melanoma: Is our prevention message correct? J Am Board Fam Med., vol. 24, 2011, pp. 735-739.

17 "FRIDAY LEUKEMIA"

IT MUST BE THE WORST day of our life when we or a loved one receive a devastating diagnosis such as leukemia. These days, outcomes are more favourable for people with acute leukemia, particularly children, but this disease is still a life-threatening event and a life-altering experience.

I have always remarked on how frequently these dramatic encounters with patients and their loved ones occur on a Friday. Maybe it's just life. For instance, we always hit the supermarket when the lines are busiest, or I always visit the library on the day when they close early.

You can surmise that the admission and diagnoses on a Friday are due to only skeleton services being available at weekends and the need to wrap decisions on a Friday. However, after decades of care and consoling of these families, it's no coincidence that my weekends have been filled with these family conferences after diagnoses on a Friday.

In 2010, a group of German oncologists published an article called "Friday Leukemia" in a journal of research in blood disorders. This group of cancer specialists reviewed 197 cases of leukemia over three and a half years. They looked back at these cases, and found that 23 percent were admitted and diagnosed on a Friday. The next closest day of admission was Monday, at 16.8 percent.

The German oncologists further analyzed their cohort of the Friday folks as to their outcomes. The conclusions they drew were that this group did not have any significant difference in disease type and their outcomes did not differ from people diagnosed on other days of the week.

Were there differences in the outcomes, there might have been an argument for assigning a sub-classification to the Friday Leukemia group!

Robinson Crusoe, after all, named his desert island companion Man Friday because this was the day the man saved his life. Could there be more to this Friday "myth"?

REFERENCE

Wilop, S., O. Galm, L. Thompson, R. Osieka, T.H. Brummendorf, E. Jost. Friday leukemia. Blood, vol. 115, no. 4, January 2010.

WE ARE WHAT WE EAT

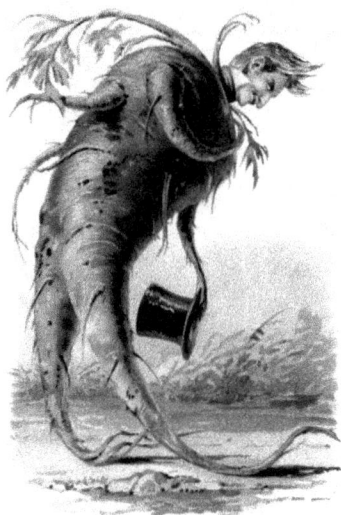

18 CRANBERRY JUICE PREVENTS URINARY INFECTIONS

OF THE COUNTLESS women who have suffered from recurring urinary tract infections, many will tell you that their grandmother, or better still, their grandmother's grandmother, swore by cranberry juice as a preventative agent for these infections (also called UTIs, cystitis, pyelitis, or bladder/kidney infections).

When native Americans first introduced the Pilgrims to cranberries in the 1600s, they noticed how fond cranes were of devouring the berries. This gave rise to the name "craneberries." Cranberries later became part of the New World tradition of Thanksgiving dinner.

Although commercial harvesting of cranberries did not start till the 1800s, it was not long before medical folklore got hold of the potential benefits of this fruit for the prevention of urinary infections, well before the antibiotic era. Apart from family members, countless doctors (myself included) have recommended this route for those afflicted — not so much as a cure, but as a preventative.

So were we right? And, more importantly, is there a scientific basis for this theory? Well, it's not merely an old wives' tale, for two scientific reasons:

1. Cranberry juice is highly acidic, and bacteria are inhibited in an acid urine. However, it is unclear

whether cranberry lowers the pH of the urine enough for the acidic urine to be effective against bacteria.

2. Cranberry juice contains a chemical called Proanthocyanidin. Laboratory studies have shown that this chemical can inhibit the adherence of *E. Coli* bacteria to the bladder wall.

So on both counts we know that cranberry *could* prevent the colonization of the bladder with bacteria. The question is — does it?

The trouble is that we don't know how much cranberry, at what concentration, and over what period of time is necessary to inhibit bacterial growth properly. We don't really have good studies showing the degree of acidity achieved by a glass of cranberry juice. Some studies are done with a juice concentrate and some with a cranberry capsule.

There have been multiple trials on this question, many fraught with dropouts and low numbers. Many trials were also not placebo controlled. In 2007, a review concluded that cranberry was effective in decreasing the number of UTIs in women over a 12-month period. Our friends at the Cochrane database concluded that there was some evidence to support the use of cranberry for prevention of UTIs, but they called for standardization of dosage and method of administration. An update on that review in 2012 reversed the conclusion. And then a year later, in 2013, a report of meta-analysis from the Cleveland Clinic concluded that cranberries reduced the occurrence of UTIs in women with recurrent UTIs, compared to a placebo.

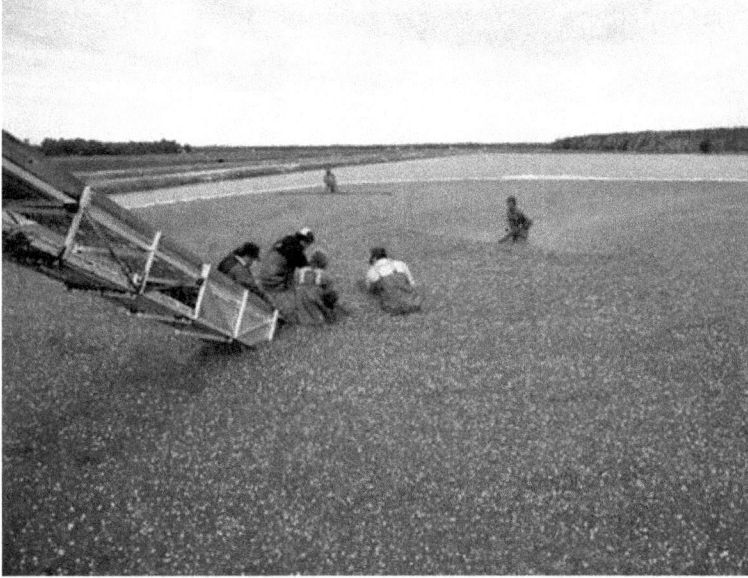

Cranberry fields forever?

We still need a more definitive study. This study should involve women of comparable age and medical condition, with a defined dose of cranberry, compared to a placebo.

So where does all this leave us?

Well, in patients with complex medical histories and fragile health, we will probably continue to use preventative antibiotics. But it's worth remembering that these meds have side effects and allergy profiles and will stop helping the patient as soon as they are discontinued.

Cranberry is safe and pleasant to drink, and it may well be effective if used by the 60 percent of women who experience cystitis (milder lower urinary tract infections). Therefore, if you are one of this group and you have a choice between drinking apple, orange, or cranberry juice, I think you know what my advice will be.

You may therefore wish to categorize this myth as a believable one!

REFERENCES

Craig, J., R. Jepson. Cranberries for preventing urinary tract infections. Cochrane Renal Group Intervention Review. Published online, 23 January 2008. http://www.cochrane.org/CD001321/RENAL_cranberries-for-preventing-urinary-tract-infections.

Mathers, M.J., F. Von Runstedt, A.S. Brandt, M. Konig, D.A. Lazica, S. Roth. Myth or truth: Cranberry juice for prophylaxis and treatment of recurrent urinary tract infections. Urologe A, vol. 48, no. 10, 2009, pp. 1203-1z

19 DOES EATING CHOCOLATE CAUSE ACNE?

IN MEDICAL SCHOOL LECTURES on adolescent medicine, one talk was labelled the "Sex and Pimples" lecture, trivializing a condition that is the bane of many teenagers' lives. Tending to strike somewhere between 14 and 18 years of age, this affliction has troubled the lives of countless self-conscious young people in the years transitioning to adult life. Even the medical name of this condition — *Acne Vulgaris* — is enough to destroy the self-esteem of any young teen.

Many sufferers report being abused or bullied because of their acne. Such is the anguish of affected teens that up to 20 percent report that they have considered suicide.

A controversial drug for acne, called Accutane, has been associated with an increase in attempted suicide. The claim is hard to substantiate, as those taking Accutane were the group worst affected by acne and were more likely to have been suicidal before starting the medication.

Popular culture frequently looks for a cause in the lifestyle of these young folk. "It's that awful fast food, and poor hygiene." However, we have studies now that show that the consumption of burgers, fries, and chocolate have no impact on acne.

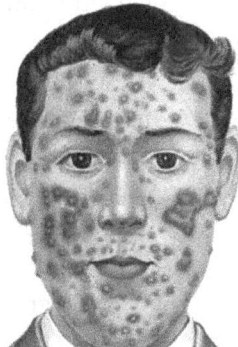

Likewise, washing one's face too often may actually worsen acne.

At some point in our lives, 75 percent of us suffer from acne. One-quarter of those affected have severe acne. In teenage life, boys are more commonly affected, while in adult life, women are more commonly affected.

We know that there are two verified mechanisms in the causation of acne:

1. An increase in sebum, which is under the control of androgens. Sebum is that oily fluid secreted by the sebaceous glands. Girls secrete androgens as well as estrogens in puberty. In women, the balance between androgen and estrogen (with estrogen fluctuations) can cause similar acne problems in later adult life.
2. Colonization of the sebaceous ducts by the acne bacterium (*Propionibacterium Acnes*).

While androgens, not chocolate, cause acne, there have been reports of high dairy intake being associated with worsening of acne.

Overall, the prognosis for acne is good. Topical creams and oral medication mean that it is no longer necessary for young people to suffer the physical and mental health consequences of acne. These days, the aim should be to avoid the physical and psychological scars of teenage years as much as possible.

REFERENCE

Pappas, A. The relationship of acne and diet: A review. Dermato-Endocrinology, vol. 1, no. 5, pp. 262-267.

20 IS THE BEST HEART DIET
AN ULTRA LOW FAT DIET?

PERHAPS THE TITLE of this chapter should refer to a low *fad* rather than low *fat* diet being best for our health.

Some years ago I heard a New York cardiologist speaking at a medical meeting. The topic was "Nutritional Aspects of Heart Disease." The speaker stood on the podium for only a short time and repeated, "Eat less, eat less, eat less." His talk was not well received by his colleagues, and the physician in question was ultimately sanctioned by his regulatory body for contempt.

But think about it. Had he stood up for 40 minutes, and showed graphs, histograms, and models of cholesterol molecules, he would have been praised effusively. A week later, most people would have forgotten what he had said. Instead, we are still talking about the event years later. The cardiologist was frustrated with seeing overweight middle-aged patients, all day, every day, whose problem was the amount they ate rather than the content of their diet. Oversized portions have invaded our culture and our hearts.

For more than half a century, the conventional wisdom among nutritionists and public health officials was that fat is Dietary Enemy No. 1. The fact is, we actually need fats in our diet. These include mono-unsaturated fats, as found in olive oil and avocados, and some poly-unsaturated fats, as found in fish and walnuts.

While studies show that reduced saturated fat intake (butter, meat fat) lowers the amount of LDL (bad cholesterol) in the blood, the research needs to be evaluated in the context of what we replace saturated fats with. Generally, if we replace the saturated fats in our diet with unsaturated plant-source fats that are usually liquid at room temperature, we benefit by reducing our levels of LDL cholesterol and reducing our chances of experiencing cardiovascular disease. However, if this dietary change is combined with a higher carbohydrate intake (particularly refined carbs), this can lead to insulin resistance, Type 2 diabetes, and increased atherosclerotic heart disease.

So it's worth remembering that, first, the amount we eat will ultimately determine the health of our heart. And second, fat is not necessarily Dietary Enemy No. 1. When nutritionalists say "balanced diet," they indeed mean balanced in all directions, not just substituting one set of molecules for another!

REFERENCES

Krauss, R., F. Hu, P. Siri-Tarino. Saturated fat, carbohydrate, and cardiovascular disease. Am J ClinNutr, vol. 91, no. 3, 2010, pp. 502–509.

Lundell, D. Heart surgeon speaks out on what really causes heart disease. Health and Wellness, March 2012. https://www.sott.net/article/242516-Heart-surgeon-speaks-out-on-what-really-causes-heart-disease.

21 SHOULD WE ALL BE ON GLUTEN-FREE DIETS?

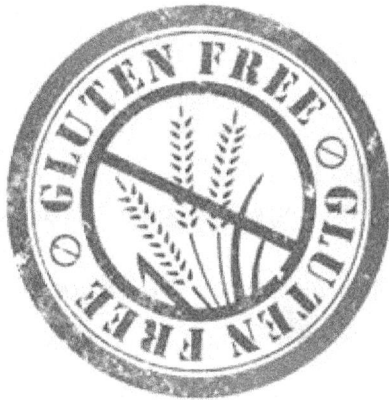

IS GLUTEN SENSITIVITY a new epidemic or a myth? Some of us would say both!

Celiac disease, a gastrointestinal absorption impairment, was first described in 250 AD in Cappadocia in ancient Greece, by Aretaeus, a renowned follower of Hippocrates although he lived a few centuries later. But it wasn't until 1952 that a Dutch pediatrician linked the symptoms of sufferers of this condition to wheat proteins. We then knew that gluten, a fragment of wheat, could cause damage to the lining of the small bowel, and that removing wheat from the diet could lead to a remarkable remission of symptoms, particularly chronic diarrhoea and weight loss.

Nowadays, celiac disease (gluten enteropathy) is readily diagnosable through a blood test for celiac antibodies and confirmed with a small bowel biopsy, done usually with a scope. In most western countries, the incidence of the disease is less than 1 percent. However, on the Celtic fringe (western Scotland, Ireland, and Brittany), the incidence is much higher. In persons who have Type 1 diabetes, it's 8 percent, a very high figure suggesting that, like diabetes, celiac disease is probably an autoimmune disorder — a condition in which the body's immune system attacks its own healthy cells.

Numerous books have been written describing the role of gluten in everything from sports performance to memory loss, depression, and autism. In the past 15 years, a multi-billion dollar industry has built up around "gluten sensitivity" and the benefits of a gluten-free diet. Gluten-free products range from bread to restaurant meals and beer. Some studies report people feeling better mentally and emotionally on a gluten-free diet. These include people without celiac disease, leading to the concept of another condition (six times more common), called Non-Celiac Gluten Sensitivity (NCGS). Science is saying that these people don't have medically proven celiac disease, yet their symptoms are very similar to the classic symptoms of gluten intolerance.

So if 1 percent of Canadians have celiac disease and 30 percent of us are avoiding gluten, are we medics missing something?

In 2011, a symposium of gastroenterologists in Oslo set about defining NCGS and determining the terminology to define it as a separate entity. A landmark article by three gastroenterologists in Italy published in the *World Journal of Gastroenterology* in 2015 suggested diagnostic and treatment criteria for this group. In essence, these people may be sensitive to some other component of wheat. Remember, we have only been eating wheat for 10,000 years — a short time in human evolution.

As to the validity of gluten-induced behavioural changes, research is at an exploratory stage. It is far more difficult to define and quantify mental health symptoms than gastro-intestinal complaints. Many parents of children with autism are following the GFCF diet, which is both gluten-free and casein-free (casein is dairy protein). While there is a lack of scientific evidence to support any benefit for children with autism, there are anecdotal descriptions of improvements in behaviours from parents who have used this diet. So, given the lack of options for these parents, should they not give the GFCF diet a try?

Well, there are practical issues when it comes to adherence to any diet. Firstly, youngsters on the autism spectrum are among the most difficult children to nourish. Swallowing immaturity and extreme food aversions are common. Combine this with the fact that a GFCF diet involves eliminating most bread and grain products — pasta, cereals, and pizza, for example — and much dairy-related nourishment, and you may have a problem with providing the basics of the four food groups to any child. Supplementation can make up for the lack of some nutrients, but not for the lost calories.

For my part, I'm grateful to the industry for manufacturing gluten-free products, as it significantly improves the available choices and quality of life for many — be that 1 percent or 30 percent of the population.

REFERENCES

Elli, L., L. Roncoroni, M.T. Bardella. Non-celiac gluten sensitivity: Time for sifting the grain. World J Gastroenterol vol. 21, no. 7, 2015, pp. 8221-8226.

Cronin, C.C., and F. Shanahan. Why is celiac disease so common in Ireland? PerspectBiol Med, vol. 44, no. 3, 2001, pp. 342-352.

Peters, S.L., J.R. Biesiekierski, G.W. Yelland, J.G. Muir, P.R. Gibson. Gluten may cause depression in subjects with non celiac gluten sensitivity. Aliment PharmacolTher, vol. 39, no. 10, 2014, pp. 1104-1112.

MEDICAL CONTROVERSIES

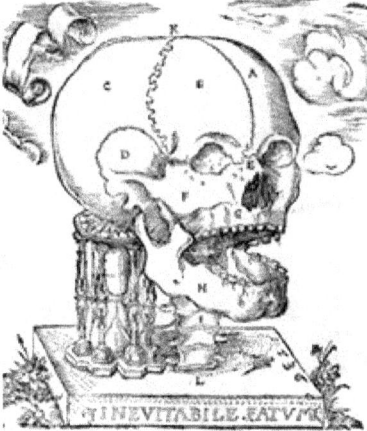

22 PLACEBO: IS A "DUMMY PILL" ETHICAL?

BACK TO LATIN again. The word *placebo* in that language means "I will please."

It can be used in two contexts:

1. A harmless pill, medicine, or procedure prescribed more for the psychological benefit of the patient than for any proven medical effect.
2. A substance (often a pill) used in a randomized controlled trial designed to test the efficacy of medical treatments (usually a new drug). In this context, the placebo is given to participants who do not know whether they are receiving the active drug, or a "dummy" drug — the placebo. To prove a medicine is effective, a pharmaceutical company must show not only that their drug has the desired effects, but that these effects are significantly greater than those of the placebo (dummy drug) group.

Although placebos have been described in the medical literature for more than 200 years, they have probably been around since the dawn of medicine. Perhaps the three biggest questions on this topic are:

1. Do placebos actually work?
2. Whether they do or not, is it ethical for a doctor to take part in such deception?
3. Is there a placebo component to most treatments?

So great is the scope of this topic that Professor Ted Kaptchuk of Harvard Medical School has spent the last few years as director of the Harvard-wide program in Placebo Studies. Along with his colleagues, he has been able to study the impact of placebos in various illnesses, and the neuro-biological, psychological, and cultural basis for the effect.

Do placebos work? Let's start with the fact that clinical trials commonly report 30 percent of respondents benefiting from the placebo drug. (Obviously, the respondents were unaware that they were taking a placebo at the time.) When we add to this that the placebo is not going to produce any side effects, we can see why Professor Kaptchuk's research is so important. His work at Harvard has determined that placebo treatments (with no active chemical) can stimulate real physiological responses. These include changes in heart rate and blood pressure, and even chemical activity within the brain in cases involving pain, depression, and anxiety.

But what is the basis of these physiological changes? Are they based on emotions, faith, or the perception of the caring physician? More importantly, are there certain people who are susceptible to placebo responses, and can they be identified? (Similar arguments apply to hypnosis.)

Is it ethical, then, for a doctor to prescribe a placebo or dummy pill? Not without the consent of the patient! In the case of clinical trials, however, the experimental subject signs a consent that clearly states that one of the blind treatments will be a sugar pill or dummy medicine. This is to protect the patients from accidental reports of new medications.

What if we were to *tell* patients that we proposed to give them a placebo to treat their symptoms? Until recently, the deceptive nature of placebo treatments was felt to be an insurmountable ethical barrier to their use. However, in the case of irritable bowel syndrome, a condition of chronic abdominal pain, and of constipation or diarrhoea, two studies have shown open-label placebo to be equal or more effective than the main drug available to treat the disease. Placebo response in one study was 59 percent. So will patients accept the use of a placebo if they are shown evidence that it is effective? Maybe!

And lastly, do all or most medications have a combination of biochemical and placebo effects? This must be true in everyday practice. Differences of only one or two percentage points have been found in some studies comparing anti-depressant use to placebo. Also, the relief resulting from being prescribed an antibiotic for a winter respiratory infection must be part placebo effect, as it's estimated that 80 percent of these infections are caused by viruses, which are unresponsive to antibiotics.

The ultimate answers will probably involve the identi-fication of "responders" and "non-responders."

REFERENCES

Kirsch, I. The placebo effect has come of age. Journal of Mind-Body Regulation, vol. 1, no. 2, June 2011, pp. 106-109.

Kienle, G.S., et al. The powerful placebo effect: Fact or fiction. Jclin Epidemiol, vol. 50, no. 12, 1997, pp. 1311-1318.

Feinberg, C. The placebo phenomenon. Harvard Magazine, January 2013, pp. 1-10.
http://harvardmagazine.com/2013/01/the-placebo-phenomenon.

23 THE HIGH COST OF DYING

IT IS NO MYTH that all of us are going to die at some point. But are exorbitant end-of-life costs a myth or a reality?

The picture of one's last days spent attached to a machine, undergoing a thousand tests, is more and more familiar these days. In an age of awareness of health spending, it's common to see headlines like "60 percent of health dollars used in last six months of life," or "1 percent of population using 30 percent of health budget."

If health policy analysts tell us that 60 percent of this budget is being spent on persons in the last six or twelve months of their life, could they be correct? Could it be, then, that the rest of us are collectively left with 40 percent — less than half the pot?

One of the problems with this topic is that the headlines are coming from different health centres in different countries with diverse demographics and variable cultural and legal challenges. The staff at Nuffield Trust in London's West End were not convinced of these figures and thought that they were in fact a myth. They decided to add up care costs in their population over the 90 days that preceded death. In their study of a population of more than 200,000, they had 21,000 deaths. Computing the costs of family doctor visits, community nurse contacts, residential nursing care, hospice care, and in-patient hospital care, costs averaged out per person were £6,500 (approximately $10,000).

For sure, health-care costs escalated in the final weeks of life — but hardly by 60 percent. The *American Journal of Public Health* recently published data showing that only 11 to 13 percent of care costs are incurred in the final year of life.

So, whence the myth and hyperbole? I can only surmise that hospital economists may have been quoted out of context. Perhaps 60 percent of costs in *that* hospital, with *that* demographic, or in *that* ICU?

So, then, it's not *age* as such that elevates spending. Healthy elderly seniors may not cost our health-care systems much more than folks in middle age. However, it's a fact that most countries do find that *proximity to death* rather than age is the key factor in health-care spending.

We are all aware that hospital stays are very expensive and that home care is more cost-effective. This is particularly the case in palliative care, where people are able to live out their days in the home and family environment, with skilled hospice support. Clearly, the funding for home care needs to follow the patient home and not be a form of cliché or lip service.

Also, to this point, we have equated "end of life care" with "elder care." But having worked in neonatal pediatrics for many years, I know that the costs for end-of-life care in the youngest demographic in our population — premature infants — is considerable. This is another form of ICU care, called NICU (neonatal intensive-care unit). Premature infants make up less than 10 percent of births but are responsible for 50 percent of the in-patient budget for infants. Mortality in this group is far higher than the average, as are the long-term disabilities.

REFERENCES

Aldridge, M., and A. Kelley. The myth regarding high cost of end of life care. American Journal of Public Health, vol. 105, no. 12, 2015, pp. 2411-2415.

Georghiou, T., and M. Bardsley. Research report: Exploring the cost of care at the end of life. Nuffieldtrust.org.uk. September 2014.

24 VACCINE CONTROVERSIES

WHEN AN ENGLISH SURGEON named Edward Jenner discovered a vaccine for smallpox in the late 1700s, he could hardly imagine the controversies that would thwart his science 200 years later.

Smallpox was first reported in New France in 1616 near Tadoussac, brought by French settlers. Because the Aboriginal peoples in the area had no immunity, they were ravaged by the disease, which quickly spread to other tribes.

Smallpox had devastated Europe in epidemics for hundreds of years. Jenner noted, however, that milkmaids in pastoral England were rarely afflicted with the disease. He deduced that this immunity was probably related to their coming into contact with cowpox through the udders of cows. Cowpox, a milder virus that causes minimal rash and other symptoms, belongs to the same poxvirus family as the variola virus that causes the devastating smallpox.

Jenner found that scratching the fluid of cowpox lesions into the skin of healthy individuals inoculated them against both cowpox and smallpox. From his insight came the concept of *innoculation*, in which the serum of recovered patients contained a substance that could protect others from that disease.

And so....

The Pertussis (Whooping Cough) Vaccine Controversy

I arrived in Liverpool in 1978 to train as a pediatrician. Merseyside had Britain's second-biggest children's hospital, known as Alder Hey Children's Hospital. With 800 beds, it served an area of several million people in north England and Wales. Its wards stretched through 26 attached buildings and rose three storeys high. The wards were labelled from A all the way to Z — the ward where we resident junior doctors slept, if such a chance arose.

Distance within the hospital was complicated by the fact that the Casualty or Emergency Department was on A ward, and thus one mile from the doctors' sleeping quarters. A hospital bylaw allowed the on-call house officer to ride a bicycle in the corridors between Z ward and A ward — after 8 pm.

D3 had a unit called the "Pertussis ward," with 20 to 30 beds for one disease only: whooping cough. This devastating respiratory condition, sometimes known as the "100-day cough," can cause apnoea (cessation of breathing), pneumonia, and even seizures. Most pertussis deaths occur in the first six months of life, when the vaccine has not yet taken. The spasms of coughing are dramatic, and followed by a whoop as the child breathes in.

Liverpool, once the second city of the Empire, went into decline after the demise of the shipbuilding industry. The Beatles had departed nine years earlier, and the Cavern Club was now the Cabin Club. We managed to get a flat around the corner from Penny Lane and settled into this unique city, still possessing the charms of its people and its history.

However, one topic was never far from the minds of pediatricians and parents. Pertussis, having been almost eradicated, was making a comeback. Vaccination rates had dropped to 20 percent. In Britain from 1974 to 1979, there were 103,000 cases of pertussis. Forty-one children died, most of them aged under a year. A second epidemic was to follow in the 1980s. The reason? Controversy about safety of the vaccine.

Media reports of this vaccine causing neurological damage led to a sharp decline in public acceptance of the safety of this immunization. The reports tended to be sensationalized by the tabloid press, while the dangers of the disease itself were given little attention.

Scepticism among the medical profession itself regarding the administration of this vaccine condemned it to a controversy that would last for decades.

But some truth lies behind most myths. The whole-cell vaccine used from 1950 to 1990 had been developed in early 1900s. It could cause fevers, and sometimes even seizures (approximately 5 percent of infants are prone to develop seizures with febrile illness). As whooping cough became less common, stories began to appear regarding neurological damage from this vaccine.

A wave of legal battles, and vaccine compensation ensued. It is impossible to tell what caused the neurological damage in these unfortunate children. There were no MRIs or genetic tests to confirm diagnoses then.

In 1981, a landmark survey of children aged six months to 36 months determined that the risk of neurological damage after whooping cough vaccine was three per million — very close to the risk for those unimmunized. The irony is that the disease itself causes seizures in 10 percent of infants.

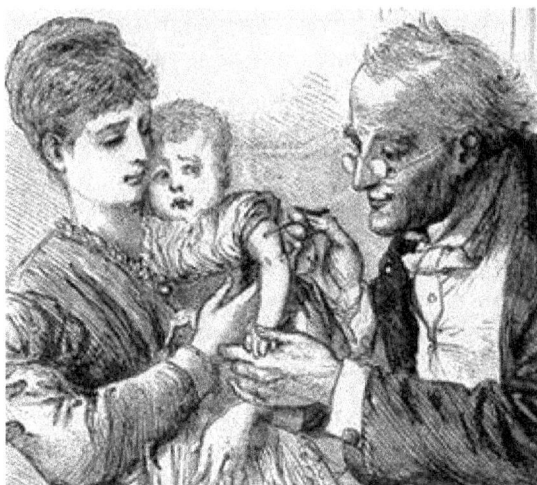

A second improvement in uptake occurred with the development of an acellular vaccine, which is purer and causes less fever.

Today, the uptake of pertussis vaccine in the western world is similar to that for other vaccines, as the controversy is now largely forgotten. More than half of pregnant mothers are accepting the pertussis in mid-pregnancy to prevent early onset whooping cough in their newborn infant — the time of highest risk to children.

Unfortunately, in the process of reviewing our own vaccine safety, we exported the controversy to Third World countries, where mortality rates from pertussis were high and more benefit would have come from vaccine.

The MMR Vaccine: A Cause of Autism?

Autism is a lifelong neurodevelopmental disorder with a strong genetic component. In 1998, a study was published suggesting a link between MMR (measles, mumps, and rubella) and the onset of autism.

Various vaccine advocacy groups showed their concern, and soon the uptake of MMR vaccine fell off considerably. These illnesses then began to reappear in our homes and schools.

The profile of this controversy was highlighted by some very well known Hollywood figures — the best known of whom was Jenny McCarthy, an actress then in a relationship with Jim Carrey. Jenny firmly believed that her son's autism was caused by MMR vaccine. Once again, very strong publicity resulted in the withdrawal of many thousands of people from the routine vaccination program.

It's easy enough to see why parents might suspect a link between the two. MMR is given at 12 to 15 months, exactly the age that doctors begin to make pronouncements on a child's development — particularly social development.

So suspecting a cause and effect is somewhat understandable — but not true. Recent studies across North America and Europe have failed to show any link between this vaccine and autism. Moreover, retrospective studies showed no increase in autism in the first ten years after the introduction of MMR in 1988.

Some of the theory propounded by the anti-vaccine advocacy groups related to the belief that the mercury in vaccines caused the autism. The mercury compound Thimerosal is used as a preservative in MMR. This compound has also been refuted as a cause of autism, but because of the number of new vaccines being given to children, it was deemed prudent to remove all mercury from vaccines after a recommendation by the American Academy of Pediatrics.

Concern has also arisen about the sheer number of shots that infants are being given in the first year of life. This too has been highlighted as a possible cause of autism, and again refuted by careful research studies.

So, largely because of these and other vaccines, we no longer need 800-bed hospitals — nor perhaps as many pediatricians either!

REFERENCES

Baker, J.P. The pertussis vaccine controversy in Great Britain, 1974-86. Science Direct March, Vaccine, vol. 21, 2003, pp. 4003-4010.

DeStefano, F. Vaccines and autism: Evidence does not support a causal association. Nature, vol. 82, no. 6, December 2007, pp. 756-759.

25 DIABETES AND THE INSULIN STORY: JUST TOO MUCH SUGAR?

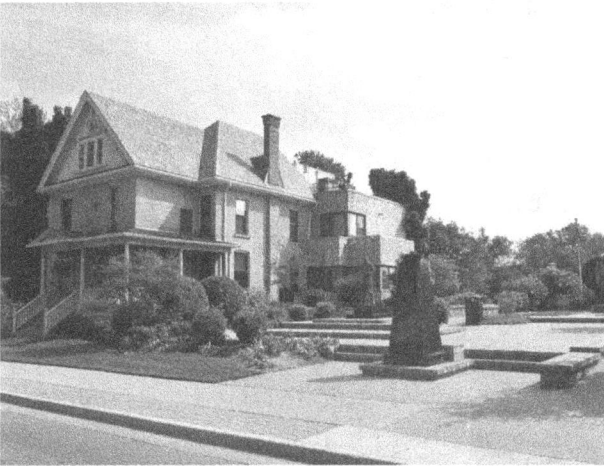

Banting House in London, Ontario, known as the "birthplace of insulin"

THE DISCOVERY, ISOLATION, and manufacturing of insulin is one of the most Canadian of stories. Insulin research has probably altered medical outcomes more than any other medical research. An estimated 500 million people are afflicted with diabetes worldwide. Since the discovery and isolation of insulin in 1923, billions have had access to this hormone to control their blood sugar.

Although diabetes clinics are known to have existed in India in 4000 BC, before the discovery of insulin no treatment had targeted the cause of diabetes, namely insulin deficiency. It's a source of great national pride in the Great White North that a relatively unknown surgeon, Frederick Banting, and an even lesser-known medical student, Charles Best, isolated this hormone from the pancreas of dogs. Their research, done in the University of Toronto, was awarded the Nobel Prize.

Banting discovered that removing the pancreas from a dog gave it symptoms of diabetes. After isolating pancreatic extract from a second dog, he was able to inject it into the diabetic dog and reverse the symptoms of high blood sugar. Dog 92, a collie, was the first live being to experience remission from symptoms of diabetes through use of the insulin hormone.

In the university hospital, Leonard Thompson, a 14-year-old boy, lay dying of Type 1 diabetes. When he was injected with insulin, he made a recovery and eventually went home.

One likes to think of dedicated researchers toiling over the research that will benefit humanity — and that certainly was the case with these two medics. However, when the Nobel Prize was announced, it was given to "Banting and MacLeod." Professor MacLeod was head of physiology at the University of Toronto. He had given space to the researchers to conduct insulin extraction, but he had been sceptical about their research and played no part in the actual experiments.

A phone call came through to the University of Toronto requesting that Banting and MacLeod be present in Oslo 11 days later for the awards. Banting was furious — the university clearly was not going to allow a Nobel Prize to go to a mere medical student. He refused to travel to Oslo, and insisted that the prize be given to Banting and Best. He also contacted the

Toronto Star and spoke to the reporter who had broken the story — a man called Ernest Hemingway. Hemingway had been working as a reporter for the *Star* for two years. He said he would love to publicize the cause of Charles Best, but he was leaving that week for a writing contract in the United States

Eventually, a compromise was reached: the prize would be shared with Best. Banting then accepted, believing the prize would be awarded to Banting and Best. However, although Best received 50 percent of the prize money, he was never recognized as a Nobel Prize winner. Instead the prize went to Banting and MacLeod. Such is the politics of medicine. Later in his career, Best was appointed professor of physiology at U of T and went on to claim MacLeod's job.

Today in our Pediatric Diabetes Clinic in Kingston, Ontario, we have 150 young people who live amazingly productive lives while being dependent on insulin for their survival and well-being. I have enormous respect for these teens who live with these restrictions and yet achieve amazing academic, social, and athletic results. One of our lads is a competitive hockey player who lives away from home for training. He tests his blood sugar level six times daily, wears an insulin pump, and maintains average blood sugar in the normal range.

It wasn't always this good. As a student, I recall that persons with Type 1 diabetes were only seen every six months. They had one blood sugar drawn by the laboratory, and visited a dietician to review their eating practices. It was impossible to know how these people were doing on a day-to-day basis. Some diabetics would be hospitalized because of poor control over their blood sugar levels, while some would have seizures from low blood sugar.

Technology has come to the aid of our clinic — in a big way. Up until the mid-1980s, we had no way of monitoring blood sugars on a daily basis. Then came glucometers. These are the portable meters that are able to test blood sugar levels from a tiny amount of blood, taken by finger pic from the side of the fingertip. By recording levels regularly, patterns emerge that allow us to adjust insulin according to the growth, diet, and lifestyle of the patient.

In the 1990s came insulin pumps and continuous glucose monitoring devices that allow hour-to-hour adjustment of insulin doses. An insulin pump acts like an artificial pancreas, delivering insulin under the skin at low doses all day, and increased doses at meal times.

Although it's a common condition, there may be more mis-information than good information on this subject than any other in medicine. Myths abound ....

1 Diabetes is caused by eating too much sugar

This is pure myth. Everyone eats more sugar than they need. Many foods contain sugar — not just table sugar and candy. For instance, bread, fruit, and pasta contain carbohydrate sugars. If the pancreas is functioning, these sugars will be metabolized. However, diabetics do count their carbohydrates, to calculate how much insulin to give themselves.

2 Diabetes is a lifestyle disease

This is a misconception, based on inadequate information. There are two types of diabetes, known as Type 1 and Type 2. These "types" are actually two separate diseases, with similar symptoms. The principal difference is that Type 1 patients are deficient in insulin, whereas Type 2 patients have plenty of insulin, but it doesn't work to bring down blood sugar.

Insulin, produced by the pancreas, is the hormone that unlocks the cells to allow sugar to enter and be used as energy.

In Type 2 diabetes, patients tend to be heavier. But everyone who is overweight does not get Type 2 diabetes — being overweight is just a risk factor for Type 2. And while a reckless lifestyle will add to the negative prognosis, this could be said for most chronic diseases.

3 Diabetes is not very common

The best source for diabetes demographics is the United States, where figures are readily available: population, 350,000,000; diabetes incidence, 33,000,000. This ratio would equate to 3.5 million people with diabetes in Canada. So, close to one in ten people in the western world have diabetes, perhaps even more. Many people don't realize they have it. Approximately 90 percent of these people have Type 2 diabetes.

The spread is different in adults and children. In children, 90 percent have Type 1 diabetes, while 10 percent have Type 2. In adults, 10 percent have Type 1, and 90 percent have Type 2.

Type 1 diabetes used to be called "Juvenile Diabetes" because of this demographic. Traditionally, children were not commonly seen with Type 2 diabetes. With the obesity epidemic in children, this situation is changing. Also, because of the genetic nature of diabetes, certain ethnic groups can experience Type 2 diabetes in adolescence. These groups include Native American, Hispanic, Asian, and African-American children.

4 Long-term complications are inevitable

While it's true that, if left undiagnosed and untreated, diabetes can lead to heart, stroke, and kidney problems, in addition to blindness, nerve damage, and amputation, this does not need to be the case, and the incidence of these complications is falling with treatment.

Prior to 1993, it was uncertain as to whether good control would actually lead to a healthier patient in later life. A landmark study from 1983 to 1993 called the DCCT (Diabetes Control and Complications Trial) showed that keeping the blood glucose level close to normal would slow the onset of the complications listed above. However, it is said that the arteries of someone with diabetes in midlife appear ten years older than normal.

Type 1 diabetes can strike at any age. A condition called DEND (Developmental Delay, Epilepsy, and Neonatal Diabetes) is fairly well known to those of us who treat children. Neither is it unusual to have a nine-month-old, or even nine-week-old, infant present with insulin dependent diabetes.

The logistics of caring for these children are very complex, but the principles are the same: keep blood sugars as close to normal as possible, without having them too low.

5 Young people don't look after their diabetes

How often I hear this, mainly from those who know little about the world of young people who must learn to live with diabetes. True, before the discovery of insulin, mortality was inevitable. But try waking up on any given day and jabbing your finger to obtain a blood sugar reading before giving yourself two injections in your leg, and still being in good form for math class. Try fitting in at high school when other teens are gorging on submarine sandwiches, and you have to test blood and give yourself an injection — and try to be cool. Harder still, try injecting your two-year-old child and drawing blood from a tiny finger four to six times a day. Yes, there are those who fall short on their control from time to time. But could you or I do any better?

While it was somewhat uncommon in the past for persons with Type 1 diabetes to compete at professional level, Bobby Clarke (NHL) and Arthur Ashe (tennis) both had insulin dependent diabetes. In the future, it will be more common to see insulin-dependent athletes at a competitive level. This has come about because insulin pump therapy has allowed for an "artificial pancreas" to deliver insulin round the clock, and also to predict major falls in blood sugar levels and avoid them. Having an insulin pump can make our athletes with diabetes competitive with the general population.

Of our 150 patients in the Kingston pediatric diabetes clinic, I firmly believe that the majority are healthier and more functional than their peers in school.

6 You can't drink if you have diabetes

This is not true. Persons with diabetes, on insulin, may enjoy a pint or two just like the rest of us. It's just a matter of calculating the amount of carbohydrate sugar in the drink, and giving enough extra insulin to compensate for it, so the blood sugar doesn't go too high. This is easier for those on an insulin pump, as it doesn't require an extra needle.

However, any more alcohol than that and a new danger is introduced: low blood sugar next morning. Alcohol is metabolized in the liver and will block the release of sugar from the liver, causing a complication called hypoglycemia. This is a state of unconsciousness that can lead to a seizure. Rapid infusion of sugar is necessary to reverse it. We see this problem in teens who haven't been educated in how to manage alcohol at parties.

7 Diabetes hurts your employment prospects

This, thankfully, is becoming a myth. An employer does not have the right to insist on disclosure of your medical file. However, if you don't tell your employer about your condition, it's hard to arrange time off to check blood sugar and take insulin or even to eat regularly. So most people are up front, and the rights of persons with disabilities ensure that you can't be discriminated against because of your medical problem (3.5 million Canadians, after all).

But what of the danger to others? This is where good judgment needs to rule. In 2006, the RCMP ruled that if a criminal is allowed to have Type 1, then surely a police officer with Type 1 diabetes should be eligible to work on the force! Therefore, diabetes is no longer an impediment to joining the Mounties.

In the past, the medical profession was unable to provide sufficient reassurance regarding the risk of low blood sugar in persons working in dangerous positions. This is not so much the case anymore, although hypoglycemia is not 100 percent predictable. Truck drivers with diabetes, for instance, have strict protocols to follow: they must test blood sugars before driving and at regular intervals thereafter.

The Canadian and American armed forces are exempt from anti-discrimination laws. You cannot join the armed forces if you have insulin-dependent diabetes. If you develop Type 1 diabetes while you are serving, you will be discharged with a severance.

What about flying a plane? Well, this varies. The U.S. Federal Aviation Authority identifies insulin use as a disqualifying condition to receiving a medical certificate to fly an aircraft. However, it is possible to obtain a third class licence to fly a private recreational plane. Amazingly, Canada (2001) and the UK (2012) have been allowing pilots with Type 1 diabetes to fly aircrafts even in American airspace. The protocol for these pilots is a blood sugar test one hour before flight; test one hour into flight; test hourly during flight; and test 30 minutes before landing.

Unfortunately, Type 1 diabetes still precludes you from becoming an astronaut!

REFERENCES

Bliss, M. Banting: A biography, University of Toronto Press. March 1993.

Fox, L.A., L.M. Bucklow, S.D. Smith, T. Wysocki, N. Mauras. A randomised controlled trial of insulin pump therapy on diabetes control and family life in children 1-6 yrs old, with Type 1 diabetes. Diabetes Care, vol. 28, no. 6, June 2005, pp. 1277-1281.

26 SUBSTANCE ABUSE: A PROBLEM OF THE YOUNG?

IT'S NOT HARD TO SPOT someone who is abusing substances, especially if you are familiar with the person. The changes in behaviour, facial expression, speech, or cognition are usually clear.

However, our perception of a substance abuser is generally of a young person, high or otherwise intoxicated, perhaps associated with music or other entertainment. Celebrity personalities with substance-abuse problems do tend to belong to a younger generation. But is it a myth that older adults don't use or abuse mood-altering substances?

Deteriorating function in an older person can be associated with progressive neurological disease or prescription drugs. However, these symptoms can also be caused by abuse of drugs and/or alcohol.

Traditionally, older adults have not shown high rates of substance abuse compared to younger people. But the Baby Boomer generation came of age at a time of great social change, with changing attitudes to drug (and alcohol) use not seen in previous generations. The prevalence of Substance Use Disorder (SUD) has remained high in this demographic as it ages. Today, Boomers (aged 50 to 69) make up around one-quarter of the population in Canada and the United States.

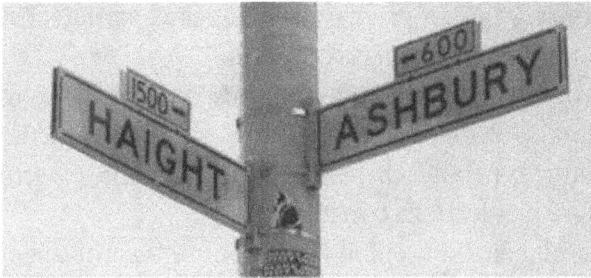

Consequently, the proportion of older people needing treatment for SUD will grow considerably. For example, SUD rates in persons over aged 50 are expected to double from 2006 to 2020.

Despite the cultural shift to mood-altering drugs in seniors, alcohol remains the most commonly abused substance in persons over 65. Although most older persons reduce their alcohol use as they age, the true incidence of AUD (alcohol use disorder) is skewed by underreporting. Current rates of binge drinking in over-65s is 19.6 percent for men and 6.3 percent for women.

Tobacco use is also quite prevalent in over-65s. Smoking cessation interventions are generally less successful in this age group because of physiological dependence on nicotine after a lifetime of smoking.

Illicit drug use is more prevalent among American seniors than those of any other country. Over one million reported using cocaine, methamphetamine, or heroin. In older adults cannabis use is more prevalent than the use of other drugs. Among adults over the age of 50, 4.6 million reported using cannabis in 2014. With the relaxation of marijuana laws and the passage of medical marijuana legislation, the prevalence of its use among this group may well increase, particularly if it is used to cope with the effects of illness.

One of the biggest sources of abused drugs is the medical profession. Older adults take more prescribed medications than younger people. Of persons aged 60 to 85, one-third are taking five medications concurrently!

Rates of benzodiazepine (Valium) use are the highest for this group for the psychoactive drugs.

So, one can see that drug abuse problems are by no means unique to the young.

REFERENCE

Kuerbis, A., P. Sacco, D. Blazer, and A. Moore. Substance abuse among older adults. Clinics in GeriatricMedicine, vol. 30, no. 3, 2014, pp. 629-654.

27 CAN LISTENING TO CLASSICAL MUSIC MAKE US SMARTER?

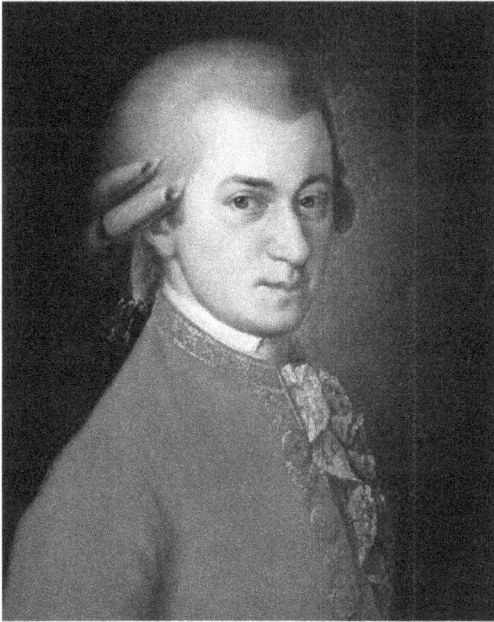

Clever Mozart, a frequent music listener

A SIZABLE INDUSTRY has built up around the concept that listening to classical music will make us smarter. CDs, DVDs, and promotional materials from Baby Einstein, Baby Mozart, and Baby Beethoven multimedia musical products have grown across five continents, based on a belief that listening to classical music will make children more intelligent.

The same theory has circulated on college and university campuses over the past 20 years or so. Could it be true? Or could it be that our taste in music reveals how smart (or not smart) we are?

The term "Mozart Effect" is used to describe a theory that both children and adults can improve their IQ by listening to classical music. This has led to the trend of pregnant mothers playing sonatas to their unborn children.

Why would people believe this? The idea that music benefits the brain and results in improvement in human behaviour is not a new concept. However, a paper published in 1993 in the international science journal *Nature* described a group of 36 college students who had listened to a Mozart sonata scoring better in *part* of an IQ test compared to those students who didn't listen to the music. The other group of students listened to a relaxation track or to nothing. The benefit lasted for 15 minutes.

An IQ test measures several areas of intellectual function. In this instance, only one area showed a short-term improvement in score. This was the skill of spatial reasoning. In layperson terms, the students did better in a task of paper folding! The improvement was 8.5 percent spatial IQ points.

It was never the intent of the author of the study to infer that paper folding equals general intelligence. Neither were the study results meant to transfer to children or fetuses. However, the cat was out of the bag, and people liked this theory and wanted to run with it.

The governor of Georgia, Zell Miller, mandated in 1998 that mothers of newborns in that state be given classical music

CDs. In the state of Florida, daycares were required to pump symphonies through their sound systems.

Six years later, psychologist Christopher Chabris set about analyzing the data supporting the validity of the Mozart Effect. He looked at 16 studies related to its effectiveness, finding a benefit of 1.5 points solely related to the paper-folding task. This finding was probably due to chance alone.

The Ministry of Education and Research in Germany then published a second review done by "musically inclined scientists" and declared the phenomenon non-existent.

It seems that Frances Rauscher, the psychologist who published the original study, was horrified by the runaway response to her article. She does, however, still advocate piano lessons for pre-schoolers to raise their intelligence.

REFERENCES

Rauscher, F.H., G.L. Shaw, K.N. Ky. Music and spatial task performance. Nature, vol. 365, no. 6447, 1993, p. 611.

White-Schwoch, T., K.W. Carr, S. Anderson, D.L. Strait, N. Kraus. Older adults benefit from music training in early life: Biological evidence for long term training-driven plasticity. Neuroscience 33, no. 45, 2013, pp. 17667–17674.

A POTPOURRI OF
MEDICAL MYTHOLOGY

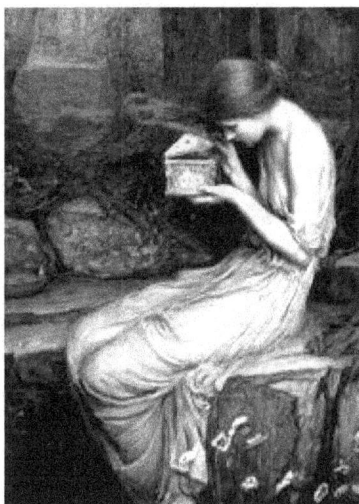

28 HEAD LICE: SIGN OF POOR SOCIAL CONDITIONS?

OF COURSE OUR children couldn't possibly have head lice. Our home is so clean!

Head lice have been around for upwards of 100,000 years. DNA technology has detected head lice on mummies in Egypt and in Aztec burial sites in South America.

Our culture acknowledges the familiarity of head lice in words woven through our everyday language.

After all, the weather is *lousy,* isnt it?

We wish others would stop *nit-picking.*

And now we have to go through everything with a *fine-tooth comb.*

But are head lice in fact a problem of poor hygiene or lower socio-economic groups? We now know that the human parasite *Pediculus humanus capitis* has no preference for dirty hair, and may in fact prefer clean hair. This parasite lives on the blood of humans and cannot live longer than 48 hours off a human body. The lice suck blood from the scalp and leave saliva behind under the skin. This saliva causes severe itching.

Poor hygiene is not a risk factor, but *clustering* is. Schools and daycares are thus common sources of outbreaks. Head lice are found in particularly large numbers in children aged three to eleven. Girls, because many have longer hair, are more likely to spread lice by having hair touching hair. Three to four girls are affected for every boy.

Studies in Belgium found a prevalence of head lice in 8 percent of school-aged children but did not observe any higher incidence in schools in lower socio-economic areas. However, there were more treatment failures in lower socio-economic groups, possibly because of poorer compliance with treatment related to cost.

So stay calm if you get the dreaded note home from school announcing that your child has head lice. Unlike its cousin the body louse (*Pediculus humanus corporis*), the head louse does not cause disease in humans. Treatment is readily available and should be continued until the problem is eradicated.

REFERENCES

Williams, S., H. Lapeere, N. Haedens, I. Pasteels, J.M. Naeyaert, J. De Maeseneer. The importance of socioeconomic status and individual characteristics on the prevalence of headlice in schoolchildren. Eur J Dermatol, vol. 15, no. 5, 2005, pp. 387–392.

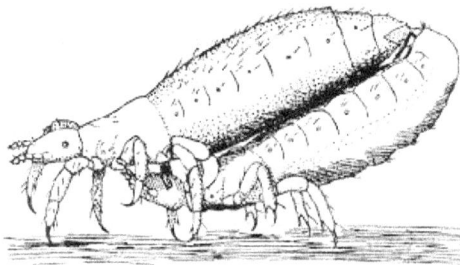

29 TEETHING AND FEVER: DO THEY GO HAND IN HAND?

PARENTS AND DOCTORS — but particularly parents — have long ascribed fevers in infants to teething. Other behaviours and signs including facial rashes, drooling, and insomnia have also been blamed on the eruption of teeth. Hippocrates in the fourth century BC described teething in infants as causing fever, diarrhoea, and convulsions.

While it is sometimes convenient to blame vague symptoms in young children on tooth eruption, there may be reasons why your doctor may not want you to believe that teething is a source of fever. What if the fever were really due to a more serious illness, such as meningitis or pneumonia?

If we are to believe that teething causes fever, then by definition all infants would develop fever, as all infants eventually have teeth. A few efforts have been made to establish scientific support for these claims. But infants can teethe at any time between three and nine months, so how would studies determine the time of teething?

In recent years, several studies have managed to capture this phenomenon. This research was done in three different sites: in Israel, Michigan, and Cleveland, Ohio. The methodology was important. In one study, 125 children were enrolled and their temperatures were measured twice daily. Researchers completed symptom data on 475 tooth eruptions for 19,422 child days. In the eight-day window of four days before to three days after tooth eruption, low-grade temperatures of greater than one standard deviation were significantly associated with teething. Temperatures above 38.8 degrees Celsius or 102 degrees Fahrenheit were not.

What these studies tell us is that low-grade fevers at the time of tooth eruption are common. However, what your pediatrician wants you to know is that it is not a myth that teething causes fever, but that fever in this age group can potentially be serious and may need to be treated. Don't assume that it's just teething!

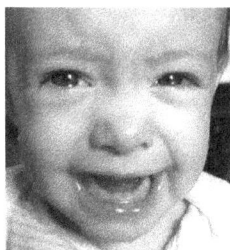

REFERENCES

Jaber, I., I.J. Cohen, A. Mor. Fever associated with teething. Arch Diss Child, vol. 67, 1992, pp. 233-234.

Macknin, M.L., M. Piedmonte, J. Jacobs, C. Skibinki. Symptoms associated with infant teething: A prospective study. Pediatrics, vol. 105, no. 4, pt. 1, 2000, pp. 747-752.

30 RED HAIR SKIPS GENERATIONS

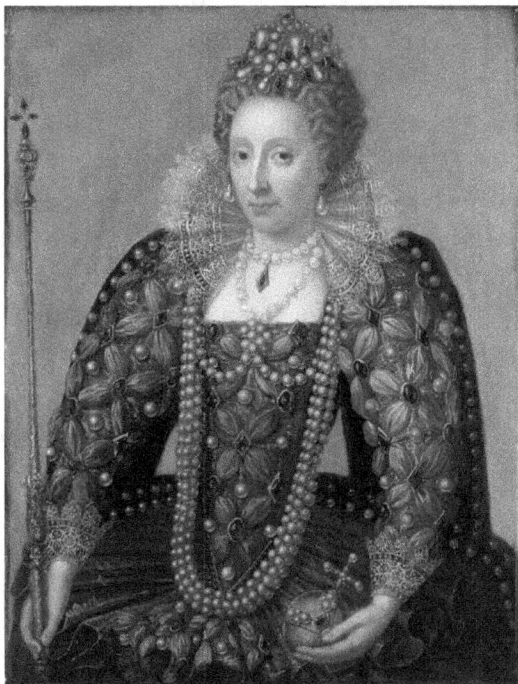

Elizabeth I and the famous Tudor red hair

RED HAIR IS THE RAREST natural hair colour found in humans. Only 2 percent of the world's population is known to have red hair. Yet many eminent people have been blessed with this shade. Vincent Van Gogh, Winston Churchill, and Queen Elizabeth I are prominent examples. Vivaldi, Florence Nightingale, and George Washington were redheads as well.

Many of these persons arrived *de novo* — that is, they were apparently the first infants to be born in their family with the ginger gene. Explanations for the seemingly erratic appearance of red hair ranged from a belief that somehow the trait just skips generations to observations that the milkman (when there were milkmen) also had red hair.

In the 1990s, the MC1R gene was identified as the recessive gene determining red hair. Approximately 50 percent of Scots and Irish people carry this gene. Recessive genes are passed from parent to child, but two such genes are needed to express a recessive trait. Therefore, two parents with black hair could be carriers and have a child with red hair. Clearly, if one parent already had red hair, that parent was carrying both copies of the gene. If that parent's partner was a carrier, then 50 percent of their offspring would manifest the ginger gene.

Oliver Cromwell (himself a ginger) deported many thousands of Irishmen to the West Indies in 1649 after the Battle of Drogheda. The purpose was to provide labour for the Caribbean colonies. Many generations later, in the twentieth century, a Canadian dentist reported that some of his black patients had red hair. This trait had apparently taken many generations to appear.

Therefore red hair doesn't skip generations. It simply takes two MC1R carriers to make a redhead.

REFERENCE

Flanagan, N., E. Healy, A. Ray, S. Phillips, C. Todd, I. Jackson, M. Birch-Machin, J. Rees. Pleitropic effects of MC1R gene on human pigmentation. Human Mol Genet, vol. 9, no. 17, 2000, pp. 2531-2537.

31 WILL MARIJUANA HELP
YOUR CHILD'S SEIZURES?

IT IS COMMONLY BELIEVED that the use of marijuana as a medicinal plant started in the 1960s. In fact its medicinal use dates back five millennia, having begun in India and moved west much later. The list of conditions treated with marijuana include glaucoma, spasticity, asthma, nausea, depression, anxiety, and anorexia.

The first attempts to treat epileptic seizures with marijuana date back to 1881. Even today, 30 percent of epilepsy patients have uncontrolled seizures, so it can't be a surprise that patients and their loved ones still seek alternative treatments, marijuana being one of them.

Marijuana has two active ingredients, THC and CBD. Both have been shown to have anticonvulsant properties in animal models with epileptic seizures. But these are *animal* models.

In humans, evidence exists of benefit of cannabis for treatment of spasticity and pain in multiple sclerosis.

In children, there is a severe form of epilepsy called Dravet Syndrome, or severe myoclonic epilepsy of infancy, which is refractory to anticonvulsant treatment. Surveys of parents who used cannabis to treat these children reported a reduction in seizures in 84 percent of cases. The children were between two and 16 years of age. The use of CBD-enriched cannabis was well tolerated.

Based on these reports, a number of families moved to Colorado where marijuana was legal and easily accessible. The American Epilepsy Society, however, felt that the reports did not constitute sufficient scientific evidence and called for more research. All the media hype may have led to increased expectations on the part of parents, which may have biased some of the reports.

There seems little doubt, experimentally, that THC and CBD both have anticonvulsant properties. These properties are dose-dependent in animal models. However, scientific studies need to be undertaken to quantify these effects and also to determine the safety of cannabinoids, particularly for children.

Most studies to date show very good tolerance of CBD in humans. But THC, the psychoactive component of marijuana, does have addictive properties. Most of our data on side effects of cannabis use comes from recreational users. These side effects include impaired short-term memory, decreased motor coordination, altered judgment, paranoia, and psychosis. While poor school performance has been documented in adolescents using marijuana recreationally, we have very little data on cannabis effects on the developing brain — especially for children under the age of five.

And if cannabis is going to be smoked, there will be concerns regarding bronchitis, airway infections, and perhaps cancer.

Yet another concern is the potential for interaction with other drugs. However, there is no evidence that these inter- actions would be any more complex than the interactions of existing drugs. Moreover, the side effects of marijuana need to be measured against the high burden of side effects from tradi- tional anti-epileptic medications.

So while the majority of patients who have used cannabis are convinced of its benefit in reducing seizures, neurologists do not yet feel there is sufficient evidence to recommend these substances without further studies.

Although your child may not be prescribed a joint for seizure control any time soon, it is not a total myth that marijuana has a beneficial effect for at least some young epilepsy patients.

REFERENCE

Detyniecki, K., and L. Hirsch. Marijuana use in epilepsy: The myth and the reality. Current Neurology and Neuroscience Reports, vol. 15, 2015, p. 65.

32 ARE BILINGUAL CHILDREN SMARTER CHILDREN?

PEOPLE ONCE BELIEVED that knowing more than one language confused the mind, and thus the consequences of bilingualism were detrimental. That belief now looks to be a myth.

More than half the world speaks a second language. This tends to be more the case in Europe than in North America. In Europe, 56 percent of residents are bilingual (in Luxembourg, 99 percent). Interestingly, in Los Angeles, 60 percent of people speak a language at home additional to English.

Interest has risen among parents in having their young children learn a second language. This isn't just good for international relations; it's also based on a belief that there are other benefits to acquiring an additional language, including cognitive flexibility and possibly reduced chances of dementia.

Studies in Holland comparing unilingual and bilingual teaching programs indicate that children who are sent to bilingual or immersion schools do better academically than their monolingual counterparts, and perhaps socially as well. So, are these just smart kids of preppy parents who would do well anyway? No! When testing was corrected for childhood intelligence, gathered at age 11, and retested in later adult life, the results were consistent: learning a second language is beneficial.

Are all those benefits all linguistic, or are there other cognitive benefits as well? A growing number of studies indicate that lifelong bilinguals outperform monolinguals on a number of cognitive tests that have nothing to do with language. These tests involve reaction time and speed of processing.

Fundamentally, the bilingual brain is not just a better storehouse of vocabulary: bilinguals at all ages demonstrate better *executive control.* These are the skills that are tied to working memory, inhibition, and switching attention. As such, these skills support high level thought, multi-tasking, and sustained attention.

Executive control is central to academic achievement. It also declines early in the aging process. These insights therefore, imply a protective effect of bilingualism against age-related cognitive decline. The benefits were further enhanced when third and even fourth languages were added.

Is it true that there is a lower incidence of Alzheimer's in bilinguals? It would seem so. This resilience is based on the theory of "cognitive reserve," which refers to the mind's ability to maximize performance through the recruitment of brain networks or alternative strategies. Learning another language enriches the brain's networks, giving it extra protection against cognitive decline.

Clearly, learning more than one language makes us smarter, longer. Does it matter whether these language skills are learnt in bilingual Montreal, in a chaotic refugee camp, or at an expensive private school? Does it matter if a language is learned in infancy (*la langue maternelle*), in teen or adult life, at university, or after emigrating?

Not necessarily. Benefits have been seen in people who acquired an additional language, regardless of how, where, or when.

REFERENCES

Bialystock, E., F. Craik, G. Luk. Bilingualism: Consequences for mind and brain. Trends in Cognitive Sciences, vol. 16, 2012, pp. 240-250.

Kristoffels, I., A. DeHaan, L. Steenbergen, W. Van Den Wildenbergen, L. Colzato. Two is better than one: Bilingual education promotes the flexible mind. Psychological Research, vol. 79, 2015, pp. 371-379.

Bak, T., J. Nissan, M. Allerhand, I. Deary. Does bilingualism influence cognitive aging? Ann Neurol, vol. 75, 2014, pp. 959-963.

33 ARE BLOOD TRANSFUSIONS UNSAFE?

DONATING BLOOD has long been viewed as a noble gesture. If you lived in Dublin, you were often rewarded with a pint of Guinness for your trouble!

Back in 1818, a British obstetrician, James Blundell, successfully transfused human blood into a patient who had hemorrhaged during childbirth. It was 100 years on before blood groups were identified, allowing safer matching of donor to recipient. This discovery unfolded four different groups in humans: A, B, AB, and O. For simplicity's sake, group O has been identified as "universal donors" — a valuable commodity, particularly in wartime. Group AB, on the other hand, are "universal recipients" — they can be given blood *from* any of the other types of donors. All of this was learned in time for the slaughter on Flanders Fields.

Before surgery, all interns had the responsibility of cross-matching each patient for one or more units of blood the night before the surgery in case of blood loss.

In my early years of neonatology, we identified hospital porters who were blood group O to serve as last-minute donors for our sick "prems — extremely premature infants. This source was safe (we thought), could be given at short notice, and did not have to be warmed. No porter was going to miss 20 to 30 ccs of blood each shift.

However, doctors' love affair with transfusions was all going to change in 1980.

For some time it had been known that some virus particles could be transmitted by the blood-borne route. Such were hepatitis viruses. A more lethal virus, HIV, came to us in epidemic form in the early 1980s. At the time, however, many donors who were HIV positive were unaware of the dormant virus in their bloodstream and continued to donate blood. There was not yet any reliable test to detect HIV, and methods to render blood safe and free of AIDS virus had not been discovered.

The situation resulted in a particular tragedy for hemophilia patients. These unfortunate patients, who have a deficiency of clotting factor, were treated with a blood product called factor 8. This protein, which helped form clots, was derived from the blood of multiple donors and so massively increased the risk of acquiring a blood-borne infection. In Montreal Children's Hospital, by the end of the 1980s, all 22 of the children in the hemophilia clinic had succumbed to HIV AIDS — never having engaged in drug use or sexual activity.

Thus came a great fear of any blood transfusion, and rightly so.

All blood is now tested for Hepatitis B, C, and HIV. The risk for each unit of blood transfused is, for Hepatitis B, 1 in 80,000, for Hepatitis C, 1 in 3 million, and for HIV AIDS, 1 in 4 million.

There are now stricter thresholds for blood transfusions. Persons are not transfused routinely, and the level of hemoglobin need to justify a transfusion is more carefully scrutinized. Surgeons now perform "keyhole surgery" to minimize blood loss.

In newborns, some of the transfusions were occurring because of blood testing for basic levels and for body chemistry. Technology has helped to perform tests on lower volumes of blood. This advance has been developed with the help of the Jehovah's Witness community, which correctly pointed out that doctors were partly to blame for their child's blood loss. Jehovah's Witness beliefs preclude the donation of blood.

Throughout the transfusion phobia of the 1980s and 1990s, we were continually asked if there were alternatives to blood donation. Erythropoietin, better known for its use in stimulating hemoglobin increases in athletes, can be used to increase hemoglobin in patients with low hemoglobin. However, it takes one to three weeks to achieve a rise in hemoglobin and so is not suitable for emergency situations.

In some cases, parents and other family members offer to give their blood to reduce the risk to the child. This is very conscientious on the part of the relatives, but there are risks:

1. The relative needs to be of the same blood group as the child.
2. The relative may not have divulged his or her high-risk status.
3. Banking of a relative's blood can only be done in major centres.
4. Banked blood takes a couple of days to process and expires in three weeks, often being unavailable for the next blood crisis of the child.

It should be reassuring that today blood transfusions are safer than ever. But what if we had a product that could act like blood (carry oxygen to tissues) but was made of synthetic materials? The theoretical benefit would be longer shelf life, sterility (no disease risk), and compatibility with any blood type. (After all, blood transfusions are liquid organ transplants, and rejection is always possible, despite cross-matching.)

Two materials exist that can act as synthetic blood substitutes. These are liquids that allow dissolved gases to be carried to the tissues. Both are experimental, and one of them is entirely synthetic. The NHS in Britain plans to commence trials with blood substitutes in 2017. Cost will be a factor, and for the foreseeable future, blood loss will be continue to be replaced by safe donor blood.

REFERENCES

Blood transfusion information for patients, and their family. The Kingston Hospitals. 2016.

Clevenger, B., and A. Kelleher. Hazards of blood transfusion in adults and children. Continuing Education in Anaesthesia, Critical Care, and Pain, vol. 14, no. 3, 2014, pp. 112-118.

HANDING IN THE PAGER

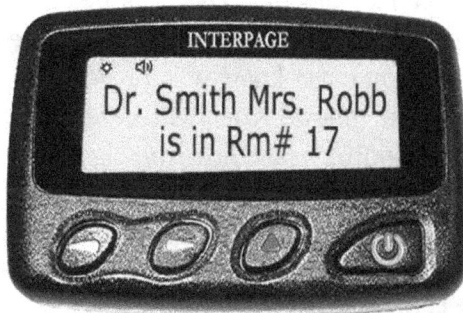

LAST YEAR IT DAWNED on me that my pager had only gone off twice in the previous two months. One of these calls came through at two in the morning, and was meant for another doctor with a name similar to mine!

At $14.50 a month rental, it was time to unload this 1975 technology, as most calls were now coming in on my cellphone. This caused me to reflect on the many ways that people used to locate their doctor over the past four decades.

In the course of a typical day, I often hear people say "I wasn't able to get hold of my doctor." This surprises me, especially in an age in which communication is so easy. Not so in the old days, when notes would appear under doors, or doctors would sit by the phone all night to receive emergency calls. And then "paging" was introduced.

When you started as an intern, the switchboard would call your name over the hospital loudspeaker system. "Dr. Smith, wanted in casualty" (E.R.), or "Dr. Smith, call Ward 13." There was no place to hide! Everyone knew if you were on call, and also how busy you were.

In the late 1970s we were introduced to "beepers." (In the UK, they were called "bleeps.") These clipped onto the pocket of your white coat and made a high-pitched beeping noise. The trouble was, you never knew who or what was calling you. At the nearest wall phone, you dialled zero for the switchboard, and the operator relayed the message as to what extension was looking for you. This new locating system also allowed you to wear more than one pager, providing respite for another physician who might have gone for lunch or a shower.

Voice pagers came along in the 1980s. These were revolutionary, as they allowed a message such as "Appendix surgery in 20 minutes, OR2!" to be relayed immediately, without a three-way call. It made a lot of sense to have one pediatrician on call for a group of six or eight, and complications over the weekend were attended to by the on-call doctor. With the advent of voice pagers, doctors on call could venture downtown with the same degree of responsiveness as they would have at home. The only problem was that the message could be heard by everyone in the vicinity.

In 1989 we decided for the first time that it was okay to go to a movie while on call. The blockbuster of that year was a horror movie called *Nightmare on Elm Street*. We met our friends, and I sat on the outside seat, two rows from the back. Thirty minutes later, a voice page blasted out details of the concerns of a parent whose baby had been operated on that week. As I rushed to the lobby to silence the pager, the audience seemed much more startled by its vocal blast than by any scene in the movie. Needless to say, I was glad it was dark in the cinema.

Thereafter came pagers with digital screens relaying messages that were confidential and were deleted afterward by the attending doctor. But it is the proliferation of cellphones that has been the greatest boon to the medical profession. Doctors' mobility has been enhanced and our availability has been improved at the same time. Not only that, but patients, nurses, and students too have their own cellphones to facilitate direct contact.

When a child is newly diagnosed with a difficult diagnosis such as Type 1 diabetes, it is my practice to give the parents my cell number, to allow discussion on unforeseen problems. Never have I regretted the sharing of my personal number, and never has it been abused.

Time to turn in the pager.

ABOUT THE AUTHOR

Dr. Michael Hefferon practices as a pediatrician in Kingston, Ontario, where he is assistant professor in Pediatrics and Oncology at Queen's University.

Born in Dublin, Ireland, and raised in a bilingual Gaelic household, he secured a scholarship to study medicine at University College, Dublin. Choosing to specialize in children's medicine, he trained in Dublin, in Liverpool, and then in Kingston, Canada.

Dr. Hefferon became a fellow of the Royal College of Physicians of Canada in 1986.

His training, teaching, and pediatric practice have aroused his interest in medical beliefs — some based more on myth than fact — which he has drawn to the attention of colleagues through continuing medical education programs and his membership in medical organizations.

He lives in Kingston, Ontario, with his spouse, Catherine, while maintaining strong links with the British Isles.

www.ingramcontent.com/pod-product-compliance
Lightning Source LLC
Chambersburg PA
CBHW060905280326
41934CB00007B/1187